"A world without tomatoes is like a string quartet
without violins."

Laurie Colwin, *Home Cooking*

Starting with a Quart of Tomatoes

Starting with a Quart of Tomatoes

Rosemary Reeve

Horizon
Springville, Utah

ISBN 13: 978-0-88290-964-6

Published by Horizon, an imprint of Cedar Fort, Inc., 2373 W. 700 S., Springville, UT 84663
Distributed by Cedar Fort, Inc. www.cedarfort.com

LIBRARY OF CONGRESS CATALOGING-IN-PUBLICATION DATA

Reeve, Rosemary.
  Starting with a quart of tomatoes / Rosemary Reeve.
     p. cm.
  Includes bibliographical references and index.
  ISBN 978-0-88290-964-6 (acid-free paper)
  1. Cookery (Tomatoes) 2. Tomatoes. I. Title.
  TX803.T6R44 2009
  641.6'5642--dc22

                              2009008964

Cover design by Jen Boss
Cover design © 2009 by Lyle Mortimer
Edited and typeset by Heidi Doxey

Printed in the United States of America

10 9 8 7 6 5 4 3 2 1

Printed on acid-free paper

To my mom, the original
"fussy old ex–home economics teacher"

Contents

Preface

A freak snowstorm stranded me in Seattle one Christmas Eve. I had been planning on a week's vacation at home in Salt Lake with my mom and dad, so all I had left in my refrigerator were some lemons, some butter, and a jar of olives. I walked to the nearest grocery store to see what they might have that I could cook for Christmas dinner and found that none of their delivery trucks had been able to make it through the snow. The shelves, literally, were bare.

In the sell-immediately section of the otherwise sparse butcher case, I found a somewhat elderly veal chop. I had never cooked veal before. But once home, with my little tree lighted and Christmas music on the radio, I realized that my own shelves were far from bare. In a basket on my counter, I had garlic and onions. On my covered balcony, even in the snow, I had a thriving herb garden. In the cupboards, I had olive oil, chicken stock, canned vegetables, flour, and rice. And I had canned tomatoes. Plenty of canned tomatoes.

I made bread. I fixed a side dish of jarred roasted red peppers, canned artichoke hearts, and the olives from my fridge. I cooked the rice with chicken stock and onions, and I smothered the roasted veal chop with an olive-tomato sauce. Soon I was eating a delicious Christmas dinner while I watched the snow come down over the deserted city.

It was not the first or the last time during my eight years living alone in Seattle that I was grateful for lessons I had learned at home about food storage. There were the World Trade Organization demonstrations, when my condo was in the protest zone, and I didn't venture to the store for a week. There was a sprained ankle when I couldn't leave my condo for a week. And a couple of earthquakes—the less said about them, the better.

But with a small condo and limited storage options, each time I had to rely on my reserves, I realized how important it was to eat what you store and store what you eat. And since canned tomatoes are the foundation for so many recipes, they are not only a staple in your food storage, but a hub and resource for refreshing and recycling that food storage because so many delicious and versatile dishes start with a quart of tomatoes.

Christmas Veal Chop
makes 1 serving

• •
• This is a bonus recipe. You don't need a full quart of tomatoes to concoct •
• this Christmas dinner for one, but having good ingredients on hand certainly •
• makes one stranded person—or multiple stranded people—feel better. •
• •

garlic paste:
1 garlic clove, peeled and minced
¼ tsp. salt

herb mixture:
1 tsp. chopped fresh rosemary leaves
1 tsp. chopped fresh thyme leaves

¼ tsp. fresh ground black pepper
2 Tbsp. olive oil, divided
1¼–inch veal rib chop
a dash each of sugar, salt, and pepper
½ cup low-sodium chicken broth
½ cup canned tomatoes
½ cup Kalamata olives, pitted and sliced
lemon juice to taste
1 Tbsp. unsalted butter
hot cooked rice

Mash garlic with salt to form paste. Stir together paste, half of the herb mixture, pepper, and 1 tablespoon oil. Reserve remaining half of the herb mixture.

Pat chop dry and rub with a dash of sugar, salt, pepper, and a dash of the remaining herb mixture. Preheat oven to 425 degrees.

Heat remaining oil in a large, non-stick skillet over moderately high heat. Sear chop until golden brown, about 3 minutes per side. Transfer chop to shallow baking pan and roast approximately 25 minutes or until meat registers at least 145 degrees (medium rare) to 160 degrees (medium) at thickest point. Do not wash skillet.

While roasting meat, deglaze skillet with broth. Bring to boil over medium heat. Add canned tomatoes and reserved half of herb mixture. Drop heat to medium low.

Simmer, stirring occasionally, until thickened. Add olives. Taste and adjust seasoning with lemon juice.

Just before serving, swirl in butter. Serve chop topped with tomato-olive sauce and accompanied by hot rice.

Introduction

This book was my mom's idea. Years ago, she pointed out how many of our dinners started with a quart of tomatoes. Want pizza? Go down to the basement to get a quart of tomatoes for the sauce. Lasagna? We need a quart of tomatoes for the meat filling. Soup? It will be better and healthier if you start with a quart of tomatoes, loaded with Vitamin C and the antioxidant lycopene. Just can't think of anything for dinner? Open a quart of tomatoes while you sauté some onions and garlic, throw them in the pot while you search the shelves of the cupboard and the refrigerator, and pretty soon something good will occur to you.

Whether it was a super-quick supper like Beef Enchilada Rice, or something more elaborate like Chicken Cacciatore, a lot of our meals started with a quart of tomatoes. And because tomatoes were themselves a food storage staple but were also extremely versatile, lending themselves to Italian, Mexican, Cajun, Asian, and African flavors, they gave us a hub to incorporate other elements from our food storage in our meal-planning: rice, beans, pasta, and whatever meat or cheese we had in the freezer.

At the time, I was in my PC phase ("Pre-Canning"), and I had yet to understand what made home-canned tomatoes so much better than the neat, cheap cans we could buy in the store. I particularly could not understand this during tomato planting, weeding, or canning season, which all seemed extremely hot and bothersome. It wasn't until I moved away and was cut off from my mom's seemingly inexhaustible supply of home-canned tomatoes that I had to face two realities of the tomato world:

1. Mom was right. I used canned tomatoes all the time, in many of my favorite meals.
2. The canned tomatoes I could buy in the store—neat, cheap cans notwithstanding—were not nearly as good as Mom's home-canned tomatoes. I didn't expect perfection. A fresh tomato from the store will never measure up to a home-grown tomato you eat right off the vine, so I wasn't expecting store-bought canned tomatoes to be as spectacular as my mom's. But these weren't anything like my mom's. They were hard and sour, and they didn't break down in cooking. I didn't know at the time that most canned tomatoes are treated with calcium chloride to increase firmness, but I could tell—and taste—the difference. And I didn't like it.

I went back to the Culinary Institute of My Mom and learned how to can—willingly this time. I also learned that I was not alone. In our now-limited garden space, we no longer grow enough tomatoes for our canning consumption, so I buy extras from farmers' markets and local growers. I started to meet people who would compete for the honor to buy twenty pounds of locally grown tomatoes on a hot August morning. They all had the same driven look in their eyes. It didn't take long to find out that we were all going home to can. We had different motivations: Some of my new friends preferred to eat organic food. Some were concerned about the environment and wanted to buy and eat close to home instead of spending petrodollars to have their food travel thousands of miles from the producer to the consumer. And some, like me, were stocking their food storage. But we all loved the end result—canned tomatoes that really tasted like tomatoes, lined up in shiny jars on shelf after shelf in the basement.

Whether you can tomatoes for food storage, environmental, or organic reasons, you are in for a treat when you can at home and cook with your home-canned tomatoes. In the following pages, you'll find some tips on growing your own tomatoes, some ideas about where to find locally grown tomatoes if you can't grow enough to can, and instructions for canning tomatoes at home. There are also more than forty recipes that star your canned creations. No one's suggesting that you use canned tomatoes in every meal, although if your family is like mine, they wouldn't notice the tomato theme in a parade of favorites like pizza, pasta, and lasagna. But the point is, if you have a quart of tomatoes and some basic ingredients, you have a good quick dinner, like Tamale Soup. If you have a quart of tomatoes and some exotic ingredients, you can make a show stopper of a dinner, like Hot and Sour Soup with Thai Shrimp Salad. But it all starts with one quart of tomatoes.

Growing Tomatoes

There is nothing like a homegrown tomato. It bursts with flavor, color, and juice. The sweetness and tartness are in perfect balance, and no one could blame you for taking the salt shaker with you into the garden. It is small wonder that tomatoes are the most popular crop for the home gardener.

Growing your own tomatoes is the best way to capture the real flavor of a tomato: both for eating fresh and for canning. Here are a few tips for growing tomatoes at home:

Selecting the Right Plant

Determinate vs. Indeterminate

Tomatoes are either determinate or indeterminate. Determinate tomatoes bear fruit during a short, concentrated span within the season and then stop producing. Indeterminate tomatoes bear fruit throughout the season.

If you are growing your tomatoes only to can, and you want to can all of them and be done with it within a short period of time, determinate tomatoes are for you. Celebrity, Doublerich, Floramerica, Marglobe, New Yorker, Heatwave, Rutgers, and Northern Exposure are all examples of determinate tomatoes.

The temptation of having fresh tomatoes from our garden all season long is too much for my family, so we tend to plant indeterminate tomatoes. Besides, our first tomatoes sometimes give us important clues that something is amiss with our soil nutrients or watering. Indeterminate tomatoes give us a longer fruiting season to readjust. Juliet, Jetstar, Early Girl, Better Boy, Mortgage Lifter, Big Beef, and Delicious are examples of indeterminate tomatoes.

Disease Resistance

If tomato plants were children, they would always have a runny nose and be prone to pinkeye. They catch everything, but some varieties are more resistant to disease than others. As a general rule, the more letters on a plant's tag, the more disease-resistant the tomato. Here's a brief key:

* A: Resistant to alternaria (early) blight
* As: Resistant to alternaria stem canker
* F: Resistant to fusarium wilt, race 1
* F2: Resistant to fusarium wilt, race 2
* Ls: Resistant to gray leafspot
* N: Resistant to nematodes
* T: Resistant to tobacco mosaic virus
* V: Resistant to verticillium wilt

Note that "resistant" does not mean "impervious." Resistant means that the tomato will put up a good fight, but may still succumb to the disease. Even a tomato with so many letters after its name that it looks like a Phi Beta Kappa scholar, like Big Beef (VFF2AsLsNT), may be no match for a garden plot thoroughly poisoned with verticillium wilt. You may start out the season with a vigorous green garden loaded with fruit, only to watch all of your plants wither and die within days as they are struck with a fungus or a wilt. This is why so many tomato gardeners turn to drink.

Also, it is a sad truth that disease-resistance has mostly been bred into tomatoes through hybridization. So if you favor heirloom varieties for their superior taste and interesting colors and shapes, it may be difficult for you to find much disease-resistance in those tomatoes. The Amish heirloom Brandywines are often identified as some of the best-tasting tomatoes out there, but they have little, if any, disease resistance.

Growing Season

The tomato's tag will identify whether they are early bearers (up to 65 days), midseason bearers (66-79 days), or late bearers (80+ days). Those estimated days are from the time the plant is set out in the garden, not from the time the seed germinates. If you have a short growing season, you should focus on early bearers.

Your local garden store or farm extension may be able to point you to a tomato uniquely formulated for your area. For example, the Hamson tomato was bred by Dr. Alvin Hamson for Utah's growing season, where tomatoes will be most abundant if they mature within about 70 days.

Basic Care and Feeding

What to Plant

We have never started tomatoes from seed, so if you do, bless your heart. We rely on the friendly garden store where we buy the transplants that are about five-inches high, compact, and not too leggy. On the theory that early development prevents root generation on transplants and therefore stunts later growth, we avoid plants with blossoms and definitely avoid plants with fruit. I have read gardening books that recommend removing blossoms and fruit before transplanting the tomatoes. That sounds horribly harsh—the horticultural equivalent of pulling the wings off butterflies—so we avoid that problem altogether by just not buying transplants that have progressed to that stage of development.

Hardening your plants can help them adjust from the halcyon days in the garden store greenhouse to the tougher realities of life in your garden. After bringing them home from the store, place them in a shady, sheltered spot outside for a day or two, and then move them into the sun for a day before transplanting. It seems to lessen the transplant shock. It's sort of a new employee orientation period for the plants.

When to Plant

Plant your tomatoes when all danger of frost has passed. It shouldn't go below 55 degrees at night, and it shouldn't go below 65 degrees during the day. Tomatoes are warm-weather plants. If you're a thrill-seeker, and you really want to get them in early, protect them with heat caps or waterwells, and be prepared to replace a few of them if they get nipped by the cold.

Where to Plant

Tomatoes like a sunny spot in loamy soil. When you squeeze a handful of moist soil, the soil should hold together but fall apart easily into small clumps when poked. If it forms into a tight ball, you have clay soil, and you will need to add sand and organic matter to break it up. If it won't form a ball at all, you have sandy soil, and you will need to add organics to build it up.

Tomatoes also like shelter from wind. They like being against a sunny wall or having a windbreak of bush beans or sunflowers. One of my friends is a potter, and his Sweet 100 tomato plants reach eight feet in height when he plants them next to his fiery kiln.

Don't plant tomatoes near other nightshades, or where you've previously planted other nightshades, like potatoes, peppers, tobacco, or eggplant. Tomatoes are a nightshade, and nightshades can share diseases. On the other hand, tomatoes seem to like being close to carrots, marigolds, and nasturtiums. It also helps to rotate your crops so you are not planting tomatoes in the same place each year.

How to Plant

My mom says that my grandfather used to prepare his tomato patch by digging in a load of horse manure and then ignoring the garden the rest of the season. She says he nonetheless produced the biggest, reddest, and most abundant and mouth-watering beefsteak tomatoes she ever tasted.

Lacking access to a horse and its life-giving manure, we have had to prepare for our tomatoes in other ways. We have clay soil, so before planting, we prepare the tomato beds with composted steer manure, bone meal, potting soil, and sand. Our tomatoes have a tendency toward blossom-end rot that isn't fully explained by watering, so we work a little limestone into the soil to increase the calcium. We use a quick-start fertilizer in the hole before setting in the transplant.

Plant your tomatoes about 2 feet apart in rows about 3 feet apart. Bury the tomato transplant up past the first set of leaves. We like to create a three-inch-deep well around the tomato stem, as this aids watering. Water well on transplant.

What to Feed

Tomatoes have three major nutritional needs: nitrogen, phosphorus, and potassium. Nitrogen is essential for vigorous, leafy growth, and a good organic source of nitrogen is blood meal. Phosphorus promotes root growth and flowering, and a good organic source is bone meal. Potassium is essential for fruit development and disease resistance, and a good organic source is kelp meal.

Depending on your soil chemistry, your tomatoes may also have additional nutritional needs. We've identified a problem with blossom-end rot in our garden that is not correctable by changes in watering, which is sometimes the culprit. We added a little more calcium to the soil in the form of powdered limestone, and the problem was solved. If you notice a problem with your first tomatoes, or with your foliage, your friendly neighborhood garden store can probably help you diagnose it, and if the problem is nutritive, they'll sell you an organic or non-organic remedy to supplement your soil.

There are a variety of ways to feed your tomatoes. In addition to the nutrient-specific sources identified above, both organic and non-organic fertilizers are available in tomato-targeted varieties that provide a balanced diet for your little beauties. Dr. Earth and Lilly Miller are both reputable brands that give helpful instructions for the novice gardener. Most important is that you use a tomato-targeted fertilizer, as another fertilizer may not provide the right nutrients. A fertilizer that is too high in nitrogen, for example, will result in beautiful, voluptuous green foliage but no tomatoes.

Basic Care

A bunch of tomato freaks at a cocktail party would tell funnier stories than a bunch of proctologists. Come to think of it, you probably won't find a bunch of tomato freaks at a cocktail party. They'd all be out in the garden, practicing their demented tomato voodoo designed to ensure a bumper crop. Whether it's vibrating the tomato stems to assist in pollination, fanning their plants to strengthen their stems, singing to their plants to bolster self-esteem, playing opera to their plants, brushing the tops of their plants with a paintbrush, mulching them with black plastic, red plastic, or clear plastic bags filled with water, pruning off all but three key leaves at a key fruiting time, or loudly praising their plants, if someone has said that it increases tomato yields, chances are that some gardener somewhere has tried it. I'm not saying that the more esoteric approaches don't work. My mother, for example, is an inveterate stem-shaker, even though tomatoes are supposed to be self-pollinating.

But keep in mind that at their most basic level all tomatoes really need is regular watering and something to lean on. If they are indeterminate, they will need stakes or cages so they can climb and keep their fruit off the ground. Determinate tomatoes tend to be more compact and may not need caging. If your tomatoes have those basics, are appropriately fed, don't fall prey to diseases, and don't attract pests—which are beyond the scope of my abilities to address—you should be eating and canning tomatoes from your own garden within 60 to 80 days.

Container Gardening

If you don't have a garden, you can still have tomatoes. For the past six years, we have grown tomatoes in whiskey barrels on our patio, and when I lived in a condo in downtown Seattle, I had a Sweet 100 tomato plant on my balcony.

A tomato plant in a container has the same needs as a tomato plant in your garden, with a few additional requirements. Make sure your container has sufficient drainage inside and outside the pot. Place the container up on bricks so the water can run out freely, or place it in a dish of sand to provide the same sort of outlet for drainage. One garden expert recommends filling the lower part of your container with small plastic flower pots, as they don't compact as much as rocks and will provide better drainage within the container. Make sure that there are sufficient nutrients for your tomato plant within the container. Garden soil will compact hard in containers: potting soil, manure, coir (rehydrated coconut husks), and other organic matters will provide nutrition for your tomatoes, although some garden experts recommend against including too much compost because it is so dense. Most container gardens need to be watered every day because they can't hold enough moisture for the plants.

Straw Bale Gardening

On a friend's recommendation, I tried straw bale gardening this summer, and I am now a fan. We have verticillium wilt in the soil of our back lot, and even V-resistant tomatoes can't withstand its predations. By planting tomatoes in straw bales placed on top of the infected soil, I was able to grow not only tomatoes but heirloom tomatoes, which are notoriously vulnerable to disease. The straw bales were also easy to care for because the garden is raised off the ground.

My straw bale tomatoes were spectacular. I grew Currant Gold Rush, Green Zebra, Mortgage Lifters, and Giant Belgium tomatoes in my straw. I also grew zucchini, and it was as vigorous and prolific in the straw as it is in the ground, but it was much easier to spot and pick the squash before they became unappetizingly large.

To plant tomatoes in straw bales, first you need to procure some straw bales. We found our bales at a farming supply store. Although a truck would have been handy for hauling them home, I can testify that two straw bales fit just fine in the trunk of a Chrysler. You can plant two tomato plants or two zucchini plants per bale.

If you have an infection in your soil, put down plastic sheeting before placing your straw bales in your garden. Tomatoes have deep roots, and you don't want them boring through the straw and encountering a wilt or a fungus. If your soil is fine, the plastic isn't necessary. Place the bale with the straw perpendicular to the ground.

Buy your bales a couple of weeks before planting, as you have to rot the straw before you can plant. Straw-rotting takes about two weeks, a lot of water, copious amounts of fertilizer, and more manure than a lady feels comfortable discussing in public. In my maiden voyage, I used commercial fertilizer to rot the straw, but going forward I am going to try organic means so I can dial back on the phosphorous. It's hard to get phosphorous out of your soil, and the runoff concerned me. However you do it, you want to start some decomposing out there in your backyard. So this is the schedule I followed, courtesy of a multitude of Internet advisers and my local garden store:

* Days 1–3: Water the bales thoroughly and keep them wet.
* Days 4–6: Sprinkle each bale daily with 1 cup of 10-10-10

fertilizer, or, if you prefer to garden organically, apply liberal applications of a mixture of blood meal, wood ash, a little bone meal, kelp meal, and composted manure. Work the fertilizer into the top of the straw with a sharp trowel. Water the bales thoroughly and keep them wet.

* Days 7–9: Each day, sprinkle each bale with ½ cup of 10-10-10 fertilizer, or liberal applications of the organic mixture. Work the fertilizer into the top of the straw with a sharp trowel. Water the bales thoroughly and keep them wet.
* Day 10: Sprinkle each bale with 1 cup of 10-10-10 fertilizer or the organic mixture, work it into the top of the straw with a sharp trowel, and water it in well.

Now you are ready to plant. Dress the top of the straw bales with four inches of composted manure, like frosting a cake. Dig holes through the manure into the straw and plant your tomato plants deep—at least over the first set of leaves. Water well. You will probably want to stake the plants at this time.

I fertilized my bales every other week throughout the summer. You can use any tomato-specific commercial blend or organic mixture. I also found that when fruiting began, I needed to add some powdered limestone. I watered every other day in early summer and every day in the full heat. I found that I needed to punch the hose into the straw to soak it thoroughly. I watered until the water ran out of the straw.

At the end of the summer, pull out the plants and break up the straw to use as mulch. Start next year with fresh straw bales.

Buying Tomatoes for Canning

Can't grow enough tomatoes to can? No problem! Many communities have multiple sources for purchasing high-quality, locally grown tomatoes during the summer months.

Farmers' markets are a great resource. If you are a frequent (and early) shopper, you will quickly develop a rapport with reliable growers. When I lived in Seattle, I was a passionate devotee of the year-round Pike Place Market. Salt Lake City also has a vibrant farmers' market from June to October at Pioneer Park, and I have purchased high-quality tomatoes there from Lynn Fowers' Fruit Ranch, S&R Fruit, and Bangerter Farms.[1]

Whatever your locale, tomatoes go quickly in farmers' markets during the peak canning season (August through September), so get to the market early if you want the best selection.

Roadside stands are another, somewhat serendipitous, possibility. Sometimes prices at these stands can be better than at an established farmers' market, but quality is not always assured. You may want to ask to taste a tomato.[2] During peak tomato season, you can often find people in the want ads offering to sell their crop by the pound. This can be an economical and high-quality option. Make sure you call first, as these are generally home-growers, and once the tomatoes are gone, you're out of luck.

One of the more interesting options is the community garden and the concept of the shared crop. Many cities have community garden programs. Call your local tilth society or agricultural extension service for referrals. You could either become a community gardener, or you could support a community gardener in exchange for sharing some of the fruits of his or her labors. The support could be financial, or you could just help out—whatever the two of you agree on, community gardening can be a lot of fun. One of our community gardens has an annual tomato sandwich festival.

Finally, if you really get into this, you can support a local farmer. In community-supported agriculture, farmers sell "shares" in their crop to defray their operating expenses. In exchange, customers get fresh produce throughout the season, including tomatoes. Your local agricultural extension service will be a good referral source. In Utah, numerous farms participate, including organic growers.

One last note about purchasing tomatoes: when you buy your tomatoes, you may find that not all of them are ripe. Sort them by degrees of ripeness and place those of similar ripeness in closed paper grocery bags. Place them in a single layer, stem up. Check them frequently. They will ripen within a few days.

Notes:

1. Other Utah farmers' markets are listed at http://www.slowfoodutah.org/main_markets.html.

2. Sometimes established roadside stands function more like farmers' markets. For example, The Fruitway outside of Perry, Utah, is more like a summer-long farmers' market that just happens to be roadside than a roadside stand. Owners like the Nielsons stand behind their products.

Canning Tomatoes in 10 Simple Steps

This process looks daunting but it's not. Just give yourself an afternoon to get it done, assemble your equipment, and take each step in assembly-line precision. Think of yourself as a factory. Even better: think of your kids as a factory! Last year, I canned seven quarts of tomatoes each Saturday night during the height of tomato season and entered the winter with about fifty quarts of home-canned tomatoes. I felt pretty provident and secure until I compared notes with my friend Melinda, who canned one hundred quarts of her own home-grown tomatoes. Keep in mind that it's not a race. Can what you need. Even if you can only seven quarts of tomatoes this year, they will still be the seven best quarts of tomatoes you'll ever eat.

I use the USDA's boiling water method of canning, outlined below. The USDA's National Center for Home Food Preservation recommends pressure canning for higher quality and higher nutrition, but I'm afraid of pressure canners and stick with its boiling water method, which the USDA recognizes as an equal process. The USDA outlines its guidelines for both the boiling water and pressure canning methods at http://foodsafety.psu.edu/canningguide.html.

Ingredients:

fresh, firm, red-ripe tomatoes, free of decayed spots, washed well: 21 pounds of tomatoes will yield about 7 quarts of tomatoes and up to 1 quart of juice

salt

lemon juice (bottled lemon juice is preferable to fresh lemons because the acid content is stable)

Equipment:
* Deep enameled canning kettle with rack (available in grocery and hardware stores during the summer)
* Jar-lifter to put your jars in and out of the canner
* Wide-mouth funnel
* 8 wide-mouth quart canning jars, Ball or Kerr, clean and in good condition. Make sure that there are no nicks or cracks in any of the jars.
* 8–10 wide-mouth sealing rings
* 8–10 fresh wide-mouth lids with sealing compound. You can reuse jars and rings but you cannot reuse lids. Buy fresh lids each year.
* A couple of wide-mouth pint canning jars, Ball or Kerr, clean and in good condition, with pint sealing rings and pint lids. You may need a pint jar for juice or for the tail-end of your tomatoes.
* Deep stockpot
* Plastic colander
* Slotted spoon
* A lot of ice—I freeze cake pans of water during the summer to have on hand for canning
* Cutting board
* Garbage bowl
* 2 extra-large stainless steel mixing bowls
* Metal colander
* Juice bowl
* Fine-mesh metal strainer
* Deep saucepan
* 1 qt. glass measuring cup
* Clean damp washcloth
* Wire racks
* Permanent marking pen

That sounds like a daunting amount of equipment, but if you organize your work station so you have everything you need for each stage of the process, it's not a hard job.

Step one: Scald the tomatoes. Fill stockpot no more than ⅔ full with water, cover, and place over high heat. Fill sink with cold water and place one or two cakes of ice in the water. When water comes to a boil, scald tomatoes in the boiling water. Put as many tomatoes in the water as possible without risking a boil-over. Allow to scald no more than 1 minute. Place plastic colander on a heat-proof plate. Remove tomatoes with slotted spoon and place in plastic colander. Tip scalded tomatoes carefully into the ice bath. Repeat until all of the tomatoes have been scalded, adding more ice to the water in the sink as necessary to keep it cold.

Step two: Peel the tomatoes. Working over the garbage bowl, remove cores, blossom ends, and peels. Peels should slip off easily. Remove any green spots. Put peeled tomatoes in one of the large stainless steel bowls. Repeat until all tomatoes have been peeled. Let out the ice water bath.

Step three: Halve and seed the tomatoes. Cut tomatoes in half horizontally. If using paste tomatoes, cut them in half vertically. This exposes the seed chambers. Working over your juice bowl, squeeze out the seeds and jelly. Depending on the type and ripeness of the tomatoes, you may be able to gouge out the seeds and jelly with your thumb. Place the metal colander over the remaining large stainless steel bowl. Place the halved and seeded tomatoes into the colander so the bowl beneath it will catch any remaining juice. Repeat until all tomatoes have been halved and seeded.

Step four: Capture and boil the juice. Strain the contents of the juice bowl through the fine mesh metal strainer, pressing hard on the solids. By this point, you probably also will have accumulated some juice below the metal colander. Strain that into your juice as well. Bring your juice to a boil, boil 5 minutes, and pour the juice into a 1-quart glass measuring cup for ease of handling. You are now done with preparing the tomatoes.

Step five: Prepare the jars. Wash jars, lids, and rings in hot, soapy water. Rinse well. Leave jars in hot water until ready to use.

Step six: Prepare the lids and rings. Bring a deep saucepan full of water to a boil and scald lids and rings according to instructions on the lid package.

Step seven: Start your canner. Fill canner about half full with hot water, cover, and place on high heat. If you have a smooth-top range, check with your range manufacturer before you use it for canning.

Step eight: Pack your jars. Add 1 teaspoon salt and 2 tablespoons lemon juice to bottom of jar. Pour a little of your captured tomato juice into the bottom of the jar. Choose tomato halves of roughly equal size for each jar. Place one half cut-side down in the bottom of the jar. Overlap it with other tomato halves, tipping them slightly upward on their edges so they fit together in spirals. If you have ever canned peaches before, this will be second-nature. It's the same pack.

As you complete each layer, press down on the tomatoes until their liquid fills the spaces between them. If they seem too dry, add a splash of your captured tomato juice, but be sparing. The tomatoes will give off a lot of juice in processing. Continue overlapping the tomato halves, cut-side down, and pressing on them, until you have filled the jar without any air spaces to ½-inch inch below the rim. Repeat until you have packed all the jars.

Return to your earliest jars and add tomato juice if necessary, as the contents may have settled. Make sure you have ½-inch headspace in all your jars.

Wipe rim of jars with clean, damp washcloth. Fit with scalded lids and screw on rings evenly and tight. If you don't have enough at the end to fill a quart jar, pack a final pint jar, adding ½ teaspoon of salt and 1 tablespoon of lemon juice.

When all tomatoes are packed, pour remaining juice into appropriately sized jar with appropriate amounts of salt and lemon (quart: 1 teaspoon salt, 2 tablespoons lemon juice; pint: ½ teaspoon salt, 1 tablespoon lemon juice). Wipe rim, fit with scalded lid, and screw on ring evenly and tight. Depending on the type and ripeness of the tomatoes, I usually get up to one quart of juice every time I can.

Step nine: Process. Using jar-lifter, place jars into the canner. I can get 8 quart jars into my canner. Add additional water to cover tops of jars by 1 to 2 inches. Put cover on canner. Bring water to a boil. When steam comes out of the top of the canner, reduce heat to medium and begin timing. At altitudes up to 1000-feet above sea level, process all jars—both pints and quarts—for 85 minutes. If you live at higher elevations, use the following chart:

	Processing Time at Altitudes Of			
Jar size	0–1,000 feet	1,001–3,000 feet	3,001–6,000 feet	Above 6,000 feet
Pints and quarts	85 minutes	90 minutes	95 minutes	100 minutes

I process the juice along with the tomatoes, even though it could take a shorter processing time. Adequate processing time is key to preservation, so if you are unsure about your elevation or the processing time that is appropriate for your area, check with your local farm bureau.

Step ten: Cool slightly, remove, and cool thoroughly. Turn off heat and remove lid from canner. Let jars cool in water until you stop seeing bubbles coming up from the jars. This means that the contents of the jars have stopped boiling. Using jar-lifter and steadying bottom of jars with thick potholder as you bring them out of the water, transfer the jars carefully to wire racks. Cool until safe to handle but still warm, and then invert the jars.

Let the inverted jars cool completely without moving them, about 12 hours. Remove rings and wipe jar with damp cloth, and then dry with soft cloth. Test the seal by pressing down on center of lid. Dome should be down and stay down when pressed. Tap center of lid with a spoon. It should ring or ping. If it clunks, the jar is not sealed. Either refrigerate and reprocess with fresh lid and ring when you next can, or use immediately.

Using a laundry marker, write date and contents of jars on the lid of each jar. Place in cool, dark place and use within a year.

Before you use the tomatoes, inspect the jar and discard if the lid is bulging, the contents are discolored, or the smell is off.

Soups

Classic Soup

Light Cream of Tomato Soup
makes 4 servings

Is anything more comforting than tomato soup? Cream of tomato soup is Sybil: it has many faces, and there are many ways of achieving that creamy consistency. Some recipes recommend a roux, some thickening with bread, others thickening with cream cheese or slowly simmered cream. I'm a bread-thickener myself; it's light and easy, and the true taste of the tomato comes through. If you prefer the sweetness of dairy or the tang of cheese, omit the bread and hit the soup with some cream right before serving or purée it with 2 ounces of softened cream cheese.

Terrific soup deserves terrific bread, and the baguettes and whole wheat bread on (p. 73 and p. 75) pair well with any soup recipe in this book.

2 Tbsp. olive oil
2 cloves garlic, minced (see appendix)
1 qt. home-canned tomatoes or 2 (14.5-oz.) cans commercially canned
    tomatoes
dash of sugar
1 (14-oz.) can low-sodium chicken stock
1 bay leaf (see appendix)

17

2 pieces white sandwich bread, crusts removed, cut into small cubes

to adjust seasonings:
sugar
salt
lime juice

optional seasonings:
dash allspice (for a sweeter soup)
fresh basil (for a bright, herbal flavor)

Heat olive oil in heavy, three-quart stainless steel saucepan over medium heat. Add garlic and sauté until soft and fragrant. Add sugar, tomatoes, broth, and bay leaf. Simmer 30 minutes. Remove bay leaf. Ladle in two batches into blender and purée each batch carefully with half the bread cubes. Strain into saucepan. Taste and adjust seasonings. Heat through and serve as is or with optional seasonings.

Quick Soups

My Mom's Tamale Soup
makes 4 servings

This is a perfect dinner for those days when you either haven't had time to shop or you just don't have any time, period. The optional garnishes are good but not necessary. This is a way of stretching a can of tamales into an almost immediate meal.

1 qt. home-canned tomatoes or 2 (14.5-oz.) cans commercially canned
    diced tomatoes
1 (14-oz.) can low-sodium chicken broth
1 tsp. beef bouillon granules

1 (15-oz.) can beef tamales in chili gravy
salt
pepper

optional garnishes:
finely grated cheddar cheese
oyster crackers

Place tomatoes, broth, and beef bouillon granules in heavy, three-quart stainless steel saucepan over medium heat.

Discard any fat that has solidified at the top of the tamale can. Remove paper wrappers from tamales. Scrape any chili gravy off wrappers and from can and add to tomatoes. Cut tamales into slices about ⅓-inch thick. Add to tomatoes. Reduce heat to low and heat through until very hot. Season with salt and pepper. Serve with optional garnishes.

Taco Soup
makes 4 servings

• •
A basic soup from the pantry. If you have some ground beef in the freezer, a few aromatic vegetables, and some helpful staples on the shelf, you've got dinner. This is really good with Crunchy Corn Quesadillas (p. 78).
• •

½ pound lean ground beef
½ small onion, chopped
½ small green pepper, chopped (optional)
1 (15-oz.) can small red beans, drained and rinsed
1 (15-oz.) can corn, drained and rinsed
1 qt. home-canned tomatoes or 2 (14.5-oz.) cans commercially canned
     diced tomatoes
¼ cup salsa
½ package taco seasoning mix
1 (14-oz.) can low-sodium chicken broth

optional garnishes:
crushed tortilla chips
grated cheddar cheese
sour cream

chopped olives
chopped cilantro

Brown and crumble ground beef in heavy, three-quart stainless steel saucepan over medium heat. Remove beef and pour off all but 1 tablespoon of the fat. Sauté onion and optional green pepper. Add beef, red beans, corn, tomatoes, salsa, taco seasoning, and chicken broth, and bring to boil. Reduce heat and simmer 20–30 minutes, mashing with potato masher from time to time, or until slightly thickened and flavorful. Serve with optional garnishes.

Mrs. Foster's Hamburger Soup
makes about 8 servings

• •
•   A simple, easy soup that you can dress up or down. Kids usually like this   •
•   straightforward soup. It is a good basic recipe.   •
• •

½ pound lean ground beef
1 large onion, chopped
1 qt. water
1 beef bouillon cube
1 qt. home-canned tomatoes or 2 (14.5-oz.) cans commercially canned
    diced tomatoes
1 large potato or 3 small potatoes, peeled and cut into small dice
1 large carrot, peeled and cut into small dice
1 bay leaf
Salt and pepper to taste
Grated Parmesan cheese

In heavy stockpot, brown and crumble ground beef over medium heat. Drain off fat. Remove beef from pan and sauté onion in pot until clear. Add water, beef cube, tomatoes, potato, carrot, bay leaf, and browned beef to pot. Add salt and pepper to taste. Bring to boil, lower heat, and simmer one hour, or until vegetables are tender. Taste and adjust seasonings. Remove bay leaf. Serve with grated Parmesan cheese.

You can vary this soup by adding different spices, starches, and vegetables.

The Dieter's Friend Vegetable Soup
keeps 1 dieter on track for 1 week

You know how it is. When you're dieting and tired, you can eat several meals while you're fixing dinner. With this soup readily accessible in your fridge, you're less likely to hunt for Oreos while you're cooking your virtuous meal. This soup is good hot or cold. If you like it cold, consider adding some diced raw cucumber, celery, and carrots to your bowl. It will remind you of gazpacho.

1 medium onion, finely diced
1 clove garlic, minced
3 stalks celery, finely diced
2 medium carrots, finely diced
2 cups finely shredded cabbage
2 zucchini, thinly sliced
1 qt. home-canned tomatoes or 2 (14.5-oz.) cans commercially canned
    diced tomatoes
2 (14-oz.) cans low-sodium vegetable broth

optional seasonings:
2 Tbsp. minced fresh parsley
½ tsp. dried thyme
½ tsp. dried oregano (see appendix)

optional garnishes:
Parmesan cheese
diced raw cucumber, celery, and carrots

Combine ingredients in heavy, three-quart stainless steel saucepan. Bring to boil, reduce heat, and simmer 1 hour. Season to taste with optional seasonings. Serve hot with optional dusting of Parmesan cheese or cold with diced raw vegetables.

Hearty Soups

Minestrone Soup
makes 8 servings

• •

Heartier, spicier, and more substantial than the Dieter's Friend Vegetable soup, this minestrone includes beans and pasta that make it full a meal. This soup is even better the next day. We like it with lots of grated Parmesan cheese and sourdough bread. It's also good with the Classic Cornbread (p. 77), and the corn and the beans together give you a complete protein.

• •

2 Tbsp. olive oil
1 medium onion, chopped
2 cloves garlic, minced
3 ribs celery, chopped
2 medium carrots, diced
½ tsp. red pepper flakes
1 (14-oz.) can low-sodium beef broth
1 (14-oz.) can low-sodium chicken broth
1 (15-oz.) can small white or small red beans, drained and rinsed
1 bay leaf
2 cups shredded cabbage
1 medium zucchini, chopped
1 (8-oz.) can tomato sauce
1 qt. home-canned tomatoes or 2 (14.5-oz.) cans commercially canned
     crushed tomatoes in purée
2 Tbsp. minced parsley
2 sprigs fresh thyme
½ tsp. dried oregano
chunky pasta, like shells or penne, cooked
grated Parmesan cheese

Heat oil in a heavy, three-quart stainless steel saucepan over medium-low heat. Sauté onion, garlic, celery, and carrots until softened. Add red pepper flakes and sauté until fragrant. Add broths, beans, and bay leaf. Simmer 15 minutes until carrots and beans are softened. Add cabbage, zucchini, tomato sauce, and canned tomatoes. Simmer 15–20 minutes until cabbage and zucchini are tender. Add parsley, thyme, oregano, and cooked pasta. Simmer 5 minutes more, or until well-combined. Remove bay leaf. Serve topped with Parmesan cheese.

Chicken Tortilla Soup
makes 8 servings

My friend and law school classmate Beth Gibson introduced me to tortilla soup. Beth is from Texas, and we were both far from the familiar when we were away at school. In our spare moments, I tried recipes for tortilla soup to try to give her a taste of home. After many experiments, this is where I ended up—actually cooking some of the corn tortillas in the soup instead of just topping the soup with the deep-fried strips. Cooked in the soup, the corn tortillas add texture, taste, and thickening. This is a great way to use up slightly stale tortillas. I like this soup topped with crushed tortilla chips and grated cheese.

1 Anaheim chile or one canned green chile, diced (see appendix)
2–3 Tbsp. vegetable oil
1 medium onion, finely chopped
3 garlic cloves, finely chopped
3 corn tortillas, cut into small dice
½ tsp. chili powder
1½ tsp. cumin
¼ tsp. cayenne pepper
1 qt. home-canned tomatoes or 2 (14.5-oz.) cans commercially canned diced tomatoes
3 cans low-sodium, low-fat chicken stock, or 6 cups homemade chicken stock
1 bay leaf
1 chicken breast half, without skin, with or without bones

to adjust seasonings:
Lime juice
Tabasco sauce

crushed tortilla chips
grated Monterey Jack cheese
lime wedges
sour cream
avocado

If using, prepare Anaheim chile by broiling until skin is black. Then place in a metal bowl covered with plastic wrap to steam. Peel, rinse, remove seeds, and dice chile reserving any accumulated chile juice in the metal bowl to add to the soup.

Heat oil in heavy four-quart stainless steel saucepan. Sauté onion, garlic, chile, and tortillas over medium heat until onion is soft, stirring frequently. Add chili powder, cumin, and cayenne pepper and sauté until fragrant. Add tomatoes, broth, bay leaf, and chicken breast half. Bring to boil, reduce heat, and simmer one hour, stirring occasionally. While soup is simmering, mash occasionally with a potato masher to break up tomatoes and peppers.

Remove chicken, cool slightly, and debone if necessary. Then shred meat into very small pieces. Return meat to soup. Taste and adjust seasonings.

Serve with optional garnishes.

Not Quite Ribollita
makes 6–8 servings

• •

In traditional Ribollita, the soup is thickened with stale bread. Although I'm a fan of bread-thickened soup, in this soup, I prefer to toast the bread with a Parmesan gratin and float it on top of the soup. If you like traditional Ribollita, remove the crusts from stale bread and cut into small cubes. Stir into the Ribollita about 10 minutes before serving and cook until thickened. Serve dusted with Parmesan cheese. This is a wonderfully healthy-tasting soup. It feels like it's making you strong. It is particularly warming and comforting on a cold autumn day. Any time of year, it is great with a Caesar salad and an apple tart.

• •

1 Tbsp. olive oil
1 Tbsp. butter

1 small onion, chopped
1 small carrot, cut into small dice
2 ribs celery, cut into small dice
3 small cloves garlic, minced
2 cans small white beans, drained and rinsed (see appendix)
¼ tsp. red pepper flakes
2 (14-oz.) cans low-sodium chicken broth
2 bay leaves
1 qt. home canned tomatoes or 2 (14.5-oz.) cans commercially canned
　　diced tomatoes
1 bunch kale, washed, with stems removed and leaves cut into 1-inch
　　pieces
1 half loaf day-old Italian bread
extra virgin olive oil
garlic clove
grated Parmesan cheese

Heat olive oil and butter in heavy, three-quart stainless steel sauce-pan over medium heat. Sauté onion, carrot, celery, and garlic until softened. Add beans, red pepper flakes, chicken broth, and bay leaves. Simmer 20 minutes or until beans are softened, stirring frequently. Add tomatoes and kale. Simmer, stirring frequently, until soup thickens and kale turns a darker green.

Toast ½-inch slices of bread. Drizzle with olive oil and rub with a cut garlic clove. Place soup in oven-proof bowls. Top with toasted bread. Top bread with Parmesan. Place bowls on baking sheet and place under broiler until cheese melts and bubbles. Remove carefully and serve.

Absolutely Not Hungarian Goulash
makes 4 servings

Authentic Hungarian Goulash doesn't include tomatoes—or flour. Ask any Hungarian. Authentic Hungarian Goulash is supposed to draw its beautiful russet color only from paprika, and its thickening only from slow-cooked potatoes. But the reality of this recipe is that the tomatoes taste good in there, and the flour thickens the stew faster without the hours in the pot that can make the potatoes turn mushy. Lacking a historical provenance, what this dish needs is a story.

When we were little, my brother and I were transfixed by my mother's tales about the beef stroganoff she was feeding us. Beef stroganoff is still one of our favorite dishes, even though, to my knowledge, its principal ingredient, Campbell's cream of mushroom soup, was not a court favorite with the Czars. So make this dish, and make up a story. As your kids pick up their spoons, launch into your tale: "Of course you remember the [pick one suitable for your family: tragic events/political intrigue/clandestine romance] that gave rise to the dish we all celebrate as Absolutely Not Hungarian Goulash? Well, let me refresh your recollection!"

Mealtime will go smoothly, and you'll be well on your way to creating a family tradition.

4 slices bacon
2 Tbsp. flour
Salt and pepper
2 pounds beef chuck, trimmed of fat and cut into cubes
1 onion, chopped
2 garlic cloves, minced
2 Tbsp. paprika
1 Tbsp. red wine vinegar
2 (14-oz.) cans low-sodium chicken broth
1 qt. home-canned tomatoes or 2 (14.5-oz.) commercially canned diced
     tomatoes
2 bay leaves
1 sweet red bell pepper, sliced
2 Russet potatoes, peeled and sliced
sour cream
chopped parsley

Spray heavy, three-quart stainless steel saucepan with cooking spray. Fry bacon until crisp. Remove bacon and drain on paper towels.

Season flour with salt and pepper. Dust beef with flour. Brown in bacon fat. Remove beef cubes and pour off all but one tablespoon of fat.

Sauté onion and garlic until softened. Add paprika and sauté until fragrant. Add red wine vinegar and reduce until almost dry. Add chicken broth and canned tomatoes. Bring to boil, scraping bottom of pan to deglaze. Add bay leaves and return beef to pan.

Reduce heat and simmer 30 minutes. Add bell pepper and potatoes. Simmer 60 more minutes, or until beef is tender. Add additional water if necessary.

Serve with sour cream, reserved bacon, and fresh parsley.

African Peanut Chicken Soup
makes 8 servings

A chunky, creamy soup that's slightly hot. The peanut flavor matches well with the tomatoes, bell pepper, garlic, and onions. Most kids will eat peanut butter in anything, and they usually like this soup. It tends to thicken on storage, so thin it out with more chicken broth or a little water while reheating. This soup is also good if you stop halfway through, before you add the rice, chicken, or peanut butter. Once I stopped at that point and added some leftover grilled eggplant (diced) and a few sprigs of marjoram. It was a delicious variation—a riot of nightshades suggestive of the south of France. So you can think of this soup as a citizen of the world.

2 Tbsp. vegetable oil
2 medium onions, chopped
4 cloves garlic, minced
1 qt. home-canned tomatoes or 2 (14.5-oz.) cans commercially canned
     diced tomatoes
Sweet red bell pepper, cut into bite-sized chunks
4 (14-oz.) cans low-sodium chicken broth
½ tsp. black pepper
½ tsp. red pepper flakes
½ cup long-grain rice
2 half breasts skinless boneless chicken, cut into bite-sized pieces
⅔ cup creamy peanut butter

Heat oil in heavy, three-quart stainless steel saucepan. Sauté onions and garlic in oil over medium heat until softened.

Add tomatoes, red bell pepper, broth, black pepper, and red pepper flakes. Simmer uncovered, over low heat for about twenty minutes. Add rice.

Dice chicken. Sauté in a non-stick skillet sprayed with cooking spray until cooked through. Deglaze pan with a little of the soup. Add chicken and deglazing liquid to soup.

Simmer about 15 to 20 minutes or until rice is tender. Stir in peanut butter until completely dissolved. Serve hot.

Spicy Sweet Potato Soup
makes 6 servings

• •

I love sweet potato bisque, but so many versions taste like the filling of sweet potato pie: syrup-sweet, with lots of cloves and nutmeg. This version forgoes the spice rack in favor of the flavors of red chiles and lemongrass, with optional garnishes of coconut milk, cilantro, and peanuts. This soup is also good cold.

• •

1 sweet potato, peeled and cut into ½-inch dice
2 Tbsp. vegetable oil
1 onion, diced
2 garlic cloves, minced
½ tsp. red pepper flakes
2 (14-oz.) can low-sodium chicken broth
1 qt. home-canned tomatoes or 2 (14.5-oz.) cans commercially canned
    diced tomatoes
1 stalk lemongrass, bruised with the back of a chef's knife and cut into
    2-inch pieces (see appendix)

to adjust seasonings:
lime juice

optional garnishes:
unsweetened coconut milk
chopped cilantro
chopped salted peanuts

Steam sweet potato until soft, about 15 minutes. Set aside. Heat oil in heavy, three-quart stainless steel saucepan. Sauté onion and garlic until softened. Add red pepper flakes and sauté until fragrant. Add broth, tomatoes, lemongrass, and sweet potatoes. Simmer about 30 minutes. Remove lemongrass. Cool slightly. Purée in batches until smooth. Strain back into saucepan. Taste and adjust seasonings. Bring to simmer and serve with optional garnishes—a swirl of coconut milk and a sprinkling of cilantro and peanuts.

Posole
makes 4–6 servings

• •

I like the contrasts in this soup. The broth has the sweet grain flavor of the corn, which counterbalances the acid in the tomatoes. The hominy is chewy, and the pork cubes are meaty. On top, slices of radish add an unexpected bite.

• •

1 pound pork shoulder, trimmed of fat and cut into cubes
cayenne
cumin
salt
black pepper
2 Tbsp. vegetable oil
3 small cloves garlic, minced
1 (14-oz.) can chicken stock
¼ tsp. red pepper flakes
1 qt. home-canned tomatoes, puréed, or 2 (14.5-oz.) cans commercially
    canned diced tomatoes, puréed
2–3 dried red chiles—New Mexican, Californian, or Ancho, stemmed,
    seeded, torn in pieces, reconstituted in 1 cup boiling water, and
    puréed (see appendix)
water
1 (29-oz.) can hominy, drained and rinsed

to adjust seasonings:
lime juice
Tabasco sauce

optional garnishes:
sliced radishes
chopped cilantro
shredded iceberg lettuce
shredded cheese
lime wedges
sour cream

Season pork cubes with cayenne, cumin, salt, and black pepper. Heat vegetable oil in heavy, three-quart stainless steel saucepan over medium heat. Brown pork on all sides in hot oil. Remove pork from pan. Pour off excess oil. Add garlic; sauté briefly. Return pork to pot. Add chicken broth and red pepper flakes. Add puréed tomatoes and puréed chiles. Add enough water to cover pork. Simmer until pork is tender, about 2 hours.

Add hominy. Simmer until hominy pops. Taste and adjust seasonings. Serve with optional garnishes.

Company Soups

Hot and Sour Soup with Thai Shrimp Salad
makes 6–8 servings

Creamy, crunchy, hot, and cool—this soup and salad in a single bowl combines the best of both worlds. Tomatoes are not traditional in Thai hot and sour soup, but their sweet-tart profile adds complexity and lightness to the richness of coconut milk.

This is a beautiful coral-colored soup, and it looks tropical and inviting with the topping of bright shrimp salad. I've given instructions for plating the soup and salad fancily for company. For everyday, just put a scoop of salad on top of the soup and enjoy.

Hot and Sour Soup

1 pound shrimp, deveined and peeled, with shells and tails reserved
(see appendix)

1 Tbsp. vegetable oil

1 stalk lemongrass, bruised with back of knife and cut in 1-inch pieces,
dry tops reserved (see appendix)

1-inch piece of ginger, peeled and cut into coins or roughly chopped
(see appendix)

2 garlic cloves, minced

1 Tbsp. Thai red chile paste (see appendix)

cilantro stems, divided

3 Kaffir lime leaves (optional) (see appendix)

1 (14-oz.) can low-sodium chicken broth

1 cup water

lemon juice

peppercorns

1 qt. home-canned tomatoes or 2 (14.5-oz.) cans commercially canned
diced tomatoes

1 (13.5-oz.) can coconut milk

First, make the shrimp stock. Heat vegetable oil in heavy, three-quart stainless steel saucepan over medium heat. Sauté lemongrass, ginger, and garlic until slightly softened. Add shrimp shells and red chile paste. Sauté until fragrant. Add half the cilantro stems and optional Kaffir lime leaves. Add chicken broth and water.

Bring to simmer. Simmer at least 10 minutes, or until strongly flavored. Strain and discard solids. Reserve shrimp stock.

While shrimp stock is simmering, bring a separate saucepan of water to boil. Add remaining cilantro stems, peppercorns, reserved dry tops of lemongrass, and lemon juice. Add shelled shrimp and turn off heat. Let stand until shrimp is pink, opaque, and cooked through, about 7 to 10 minutes. Drain, rinse with cold water to stop cooking, discard herbs and peppercorns. Refrigerate shrimp.

In original three-quart saucepan, combine tomatoes and shrimp stock. Simmer over medium heat, mashing with potato masher occasionally, at least 30 minutes. Purée until very smooth. Strain into saucepan. Add coconut milk and heat through.

While the soup is coming up to temperature, make the shrimp

salad to top your soup using the recipe below:

Thai Shrimp Salad
shrimp, cooked according to directions above
carrot, cut into tiny dice
sweet red bell pepper, cut into tiny dice
fresh basil, cut into a chiffonade
fresh mint, cut into a chiffonade
fresh cilantro, chopped
pickled ginger, cut into a chiffonade
chopped salted peanuts
black sesame seeds
lime juice
fish sauce

Cut shrimp in thirds so you have nuggets of shrimp. Toss with carrots, bell pepper, basil, mint, cilantro, pickled ginger, peanuts, and black sesame seeds. Season to taste with lime juice and fish sauce.

To plate the soup, place a small round biscuit cutter in the middle of a large, flat soup plate. Fill with shrimp salad. Add soup around biscuit cutter and carefully remove biscuit cutter, leaving shrimp salad in the middle of the soup. Repeat until all soup has been plated. Serve.

Cioppino
makes 8 servings

• •

I went through a phase where I ordered cioppino every time I was in a West Coast seafood restaurant—and I was generally disappointed. I kept ordering it because it's one of those dishes that ought to be good: fish, shellfish, tomatoes, aromatics—what could go wrong? Apparently, a lot. Most of the versions I encountered were so thick that it was like eating an entire bowl of pasta sauce, and the delicate flavor of the seafood was lost.

This version is an actual soup: sweet with fennel and onion, with a piquant touch of lemon to set off the seafood and a finish of butter to bring everything together. Use whatever seafood you like, whatever looks good in the market, or whatever you have left over from another meal. I choose not to cook with alcohol, but if you cook with wine, deglaze the sautéed vegetables with 1 cup dry white wine and omit the lemon juice.

• •

tomato mixture:

½ pound shrimp, peeled and deveined, shells reserved

2 Tbsp. olive oil

½ small fennel bulb, core and fronds removed, and bulb thinly sliced (reserve fronds)

1 small onion, chopped

3 cloves garlic, minced

½ tsp. red pepper flakes

1 tsp. lemon juice

1 qt. home-canned tomatoes or 2 (14.5-oz.) cans commercially canned diced tomatoes

additional seafood:

1 clove garlic, minced

1 Tbsp. olive oil

2 cups water

1½ pounds additional assorted seafood—scrubbed clams; scrubbed and debearded mussels; cooked, cracked crab claws; or skinless and boneless fish fillets cut into bite-sized pieces

soup:

2 tsp. fresh thyme leaves

2 Tbsp. cold unsalted butter

toasted sourdough or Italian bread, drizzled with olive oil and rubbed with garlic

chopped fennel fronds

chopped parsley

First, make shrimp stock. Cover shrimp shells with water and bring to a boil. Boil 15 minutes. Strain and reserve stock.

Heat oil in heavy, three-quart stainless steel saucepan over medium-low heat. Sauté fennel, onion, and garlic until softened. Add red pepper flakes and sauté until fragrant. Deglaze with lemon juice. Add reserved shrimp stock and tomatoes. Bring to boil, reduce heat, and let simmer 30 minutes. While simmering, cook shrimp and other shellfish.

Cook shrimp by bringing a separate pot of water to a boil, dropping in shrimp, and turning off heat. Shrimp should be cooked through in 7–10 minutes. Drain and rinse with cold water to stop the cooking.

Cook clams or mussels by sautéing 1 clove garlic in a large, heavy pot in a tablespoon of olive oil. Add 2 cups of water to create steam and then add the clams and cook 5 minutes or so over high heat, shaking the pan occasionally. When the clams are beginning to open, add mussels and cook about 5 more minutes, shaking the pan occasionally, until both clams and mussels are open.

Discard any unopened shellfish, strain cooking juices (make sure any sand stays in the pot) and add cooking juices to simmering tomato mixture. Right before you are ready to serve the soup, add cut fish to the simmering tomato mixture—it should cook through in fewer than 5 minutes. Keep testing until it's medium to your taste. It will carry-over cooking in the hot soup. Add shrimp, cooked shellfish, cooked, cracked crab claws, and fresh thyme to the soup within the last few minutes before serving to heat through.

To serve, mix in cold unsalted butter. Serve in soup bowls topped with toasted bread, chopped fennel fronds, and chopped parsley.

Gumbo
makes 6–8 servings, depending on how much protein you include

• •

There are a lot of components to this dish, and it has to cook a long time, but your actual active involvement only takes about an hour. The roux can be made ahead; and the long, slow cooking of the gumbo can be done over direct heat or in a slow-cooker. I like this with sausage, chicken, and shrimp, which gives a combination of smoky, meaty, and sweet flavors, but you can use an assortment of different proteins, or a single protein. Tomatoes aren't traditional in gumbo, but I like the flavor complexity they bring. I don't like okra, which is traditional in gumbo, because I think it makes the soup too thick. If you love okra, I'd omit the roux and use okra as your only thickener: just sauté it briefly with your other veggies and go from there.

• •

¼ cup vegetable oil

¼ cup flour

½ pound smoked sausage, like a Polish kielbasa, or a turkey kielbasa, sliced diagonally ¼-inch thick

1 large boneless, skinless chicken breast half or chicken thigh (thigh meat will hold up better during the long, slow cooking), cut into bite-sized pieces

1 small onion, finely diced

3 cloves garlic, finely minced

1 small green pepper, cut into small dice
1 small red pepper, cut into small dice
½ tsp. dried whole thyme
¼ tsp. cayenne pepper
1 bay leaf
1 (14-oz.) can low-sodium chicken broth
1 qt. home-canned tomatoes, puréed or 2 (14.5-oz.) cans commercially
    canned crushed tomatoes in purée
½ pound medium shrimp, peeled and deveined
hot cooked white rice
filé powder
chopped scallions

Preheat oven to 350 degrees. In a heavy, three-quart Dutch oven, whisk together vegetable oil and flour. Bake 1 hour, whisking several times as the roux browns. I like to remove it when it is a red-brown color. Some people like it a deep brown color, which is too strong for me, but if you like that, let it go another half hour, but watch it carefully. When you are whisking, be very careful as the oil is extremely hot. Remove from oven and allow to cool slightly.

While roux is baking, brown sausage in a non-stick skillet over medium heat. Remove sausage. Brown chicken and refrigerate unless you are using the slow-cooker method. Sauté onion, garlic, and peppers until soft. Add thyme and cayenne to vegetables and sauté until fragrant. Remove from skillet.

When roux is slightly cooled, place Dutch oven over medium-high heat, add sausage, sautéed onions, peppers, garlic, bay leaf, chicken broth, and tomatoes. Stir thoroughly, bring to boil, and reduce heat to simmer.

If using thigh meat add it after one hour of simmering. If using breast meat, simmer 1 hour and 30 minutes and then add meat. Simmer an additional hour for thigh meat and another 30 minutes for breast meat. Your total simmering time should be about two hours.

Alternatively, you can load everything into a slow cooker as soon as it comes to a boil and cook 3–4 hours on high or 6–8 hours on low. Breast meat may overcook in a slow cooker, so it's better to use thigh meat for this method.

About 10 minutes before serving, bring a pot of water to a boil, add shrimp, and turn off heat. When shrimp are cooked through (takes

7–10 minutes), drain and add to gumbo.

Place a scoop of hot white rice in soup bowls, ladle gumbo over rice, sprinkle with filé powder, and sprinkle with scallions.

Sauces

Pasta Sauces

Marinara Sauce
makes 4 servings

• •

A straightforward tomato-basil sauce, this sauce dresses pasta beautifully and makes wonderful Eggplant Parmesan (p. 59), and Chicken Parmesan (p. 60). This sauce is a starting place. Once you have a marinara sauce, the possibilities are endless. It all depends on what you have in the fridge, the freezer, and the cupboard. My sister-in-law serves up basic marinara sauce with crumbled, browned turkey sausage, sautéed red and yellow peppers, and garlic-stuffed green olives—all served over whole wheat pasta with lots and lots of Parmesan cheese. Delicious!

• •

1 Tbsp. olive oil
2 garlic cloves, minced
1 (8-oz.) can tomato sauce
1 qt. home-canned tomatoes or 2 (14.5-oz.) cans commercially canned
    tomatoes
1 beef bullion cube
dash sugar
5–6 leaves fresh basil, rolled together and cut into a fine chiffonade

additional basil
sugar
salt
lime juice

Heat olive oil in heavy, three-quart stainless steel saucepan. Sauté garlic until soft. Add tomato sauce, quart of tomatoes, beef bullion cube, and a dash of sugar. Mix well. Bring to boil over medium-high heat, stirring frequently. Reduce heat to medium-low and simmer until thickened, stirring occasionally and mashing with a potato masher to break down the tomatoes.

Taste and adjust seasonings. This sauce freezes well for several months and will keep refrigerated for several days.

Puttanesca Sauce
makes 4 servings

• •

I have heard all sorts of stories about the origins of the name "Puttanesca." Some people say it is because the sauce is hot and spicy. Others say that it is because ladies of the evening used to put aromatic pots of pasta on their window sills to attract their customers. I think that if you're a lady of the evening, and you have to rely on anchovy-sauced pasta to attract your customers, then you can't be particularly good at your primary job. But I digress.

This spicy sauce tastes good alone over pasta, dressed only with Parmesan cheese or toasted bread crumbs, but it's also a flexible background sauce that shows delicate seafood at its best and even stands up to spicy sausage. You can also add vegetables such as zucchini, peppers, or summer squash to give even more flavor and color to this dish. If you just hate touching and boning anchovies, you can substitute about a teaspoon of anchovy paste.

• •

1 Tbsp. olive oil
3 small garlic cloves, minced
1 anchovy, minced, or 1 tsp. anchovy paste
½ tsp. red pepper flakes
1 Tbsp. capers, rinsed
½ cup pitted and halved Kalamata olives
1 (8-oz.) can tomato sauce

1 qt. home-canned tomatoes or 2 (14.5-oz.) cans commercially canned
    tomatoes
2 tsp. fresh oregano, chopped
5–6 leaves fresh basil, rolled together and cut into a fine chiffonade
2 tsp. fresh parsley, chopped

to adjust seasonings:
additional basil, oregano, and parsley
honey or molasses to balance tartness
salt
lime juice

Heat olive oil in heavy, three-quart stainless steel saucepan. Sauté garlic and anchovy or anchovy paste until garlic is soft. Add red pepper flakes and capers. Sauté until fragrant. Add olives, tomato sauce, and quart of tomatoes. Mix well. Bring to boil over medium-high heat, stirring frequently. Reduce heat to medium-low and simmer until thickened, stirring occasionally and mashing with a potato masher to break down the tomatoes. Add fresh herbs.

Taste and adjust seasonings. This sauce freezes well for several months and will keep refrigerated for several days.

My Mom's Spaghetti Sauce
makes 4 servings

Commercial spaghetti sauce is often loaded with corn syrup. My mom's spaghetti sauce has the true sweetness of tomatoes: sweet and tangy in a rich, balanced sauce that stretches a little bit of ground beef to feed a family of four. My mom also likes this on rice. If you have fresh herbs from your garden, substitute approximately three times as much as the dried herbs.

½ pound lean ground beef
½ onion, finely chopped
1 clove garlic, pressed
1 qt. home-canned tomatoes or 2 (14.5-oz.) cans commercially canned
    diced tomatoes
1 carrot, scraped and finely grated
finely chopped parsley

1 bay leaf
¼ tsp. red pepper flakes
8 ounces canned tomato sauce
1 tsp. dried sweet basil
½ tsp. dried oregano

spaghetti, cooked al dente
grated Parmesan cheese

Brown beef in large, non-aluminum pan. Drain and discard grease. Add finely chopped onion and garlic to beef; sauté for a few minutes. Add remaining ingredients except basil and oregano. Simmer until it reaches desired thickness, stirring occasionally and mashing periodically with a potato masher. Then add basil and oregano and cook a bit longer. Remove bay leaf, and serve over cooked spaghetti. Top with Parmesan cheese.

Tomato Cream Sauce
makes 4 servings

Smooth, rich, sweet, and creamy: What's not to love? I like this on filled pasta with a chiffonade of fresh basil. When I was nuts about trying recipes and caught up in the possibilities of things that could be put into pasta, I made all sorts of weird combinations that I served with this sauce. My weirdest was probably a shrimp and goat cheese ravioli with lemon pasta. It was actually very good. No matter how inventive my combinations, my tomato cream sauce dressed them beautifully, the way a well-cut designer dress covers a multitude of inner sins.

Now that I am over that particular phase and am mostly satisfied with the filled pasta offerings that I can find in the store, this sauce is still good on whatever I bring home, whether it's a simple cheese ravioli or a creative lobster and mushroom tortellini. It adds that element of grace.

1 Tbsp. olive oil
1 Tbsp. butter
1 medium onion, finely chopped
1 Tbsp. tomato paste
1 qt. home-canned tomatoes or 2 (14.5-oz.) cans commercially canned

crushed tomatoes in purée
1 cup heavy cream
7 to 10 leaves of fresh basil, cut into chiffonade
½ tsp. to 1 tsp. salt
a few grinds of black pepper
¼ cup grated Parmesan cheese

Heat oil and butter over medium heat in heavy, three-quart stainless steel saucepan. Add onion and sauté until soft. Add tomato paste and sauté until fragrant.

Add tomatoes and cook, uncovered, stirring occasionally and mashing with a potato masher to break down tomatoes, until most of the liquid has cooked away and the tomatoes are soft and thick. Purée in a blender in batches. Press through a fine mesh strainer and discard solids. The sauce can be frozen at this point.

Stir in cream, salt, basil, and pepper. Bring to simmer and cook over low heat, stirring constantly, until smooth and thick, about 5 minutes. Stir in cheese and continue stirring until cheese is melted and sauce is smooth.

Sauces for Main Dishes

Pizza Sauce
dressses 3 thin-crust pizzas or 2 thick-crust pizzas

I like the licorice kiss of fennel in this sauce, but that's probably because it reminds me of sausage, which reminds me of pizza, which inevitably makes me happy. This is a nice, balanced sauce that tastes like tomatoes, garlic, and herbs, not like seasoned corn syrup, the way so many commercial pizza sauces do. It's wonderful for Thin-Crust Pizza (p. 53) and Deep-Dish Pizza (p. 55).

2 Tbsp. olive oil
1 garlic clove, minced
½ tsp. salt
⅛ tsp. cayenne pepper
⅛ tsp. black pepper
¼ tsp. fennel seeds (optional)
1 qt. home-canned tomatoes or 2 (14.5-oz.) cans commercially canned
    crushed tomatoes in purée
¾ tsp. dried oregano

to adjust seasonings:
additional oregano
sugar
salt
lime juice
Tabasco sauce

Heat olive oil in heavy, three-quart stainless steel saucepan over medium heat. Sauté garlic until soft. Add salt, cayenne pepper, black pepper, and optional fennel seeds and sauté until fragrant. Add tomatoes. Mix well. Bring to boil over medium-high heat, stirring frequently. Reduce heat to medium-low and simmer until thickened, stirring occasionally and mashing with a potato masher to break down the tomatoes. Add oregano.

Taste and adjust seasonings. Purée briefly in blender. This sauce freezes well for several months and will keep refrigerated for several days.

Mexican Sauce
makes 4 servings

• •
Use this warm-toned, earthy sauce for Chile Rellenos Crepes (p. 50), and Baked Mexican Puff (p. 52). Or use it as a basic enchilada sauce.
• •

1 Tbsp. vegetable oil
2 Tbsp. minced onion
1 small garlic clove, minced
1 tsp. cumin

⅛ tsp. cayenne pepper

1 qt. home-canned tomatoes or 2 (14.5-oz.) cans commercially canned
tomatoes

1 (8-oz.) can tomato sauce

1 tsp. dried oregano

to adjust seasonings:

sugar

salt

lime juice

Heat oil in a heavy, three-quart stainless steel saucepan over medium heat. Sauté onion and garlic until softened, stirring frequently. Add cumin and cayenne and stir in the hot oil until spices are fragrant.

Add canned tomatoes and tomato sauce. Mix well. Crush with potato masher. Simmer over medium heat for approximately 30 minutes, stirring frequently. Add 1 teaspoon dried oregano.

Simmer over medium heat for approximately 30 more minutes, stirring frequently and crushing periodically with potato masher, until thickened and smooth.

Taste and adjust seasonings. This sauce freezes well for several months and will keep refrigerated for several days.

Chipotle Enchilada Sauce
makes 4 servings

Smoky and savory, this smooth sauce goes well with tangy goat cheese enchiladas (p. 58), or enchiladas with meaty, homemade refried beans (p. 57). Chipotles are dried, smoked jalapenos, which are canned in spicy, vinegary sauce called adobo. You can adjust the hint of smoke and heat in this sauce by varying the number of chipotles and the amount of adobo you include.

1 Tbsp. olive oil

4 small garlic cloves, minced

2 to 4 chipotle peppers in adobo, diced

1 Tbsp. adobo sauce from canned peppers

1 (8-oz.) can tomato sauce

1 qt. home-canned tomatoes or 2 (14.5-oz.) cans commercially canned
   crushed tomatoes in purée

honey (I put in a dollop of honey if I'm using it for goat cheese enchiladas but skip the honey with a refried bean filling)
salt
lime juice
Tabasco sauce

Heat olive oil in heavy, three-quart stainless steel saucepan over
medium heat. Sauté garlic briefly. Add peppers, adobo sauce, tomato
sauce, and tomatoes. Mix well. Bring to boil over medium-high heat,
stirring frequently. Reduce heat to medium-low and simmer until
thickened, stirring occasionally and mashing with a potato masher to
break down the tomatoes.

Taste and adjust seasonings. Cool slightly and purée in batches
in a blender. This sauce freezes well for several months and will keep
refrigerated for several days.

Main Dishes

As Basic as It Gets

My mom likes home-canned tomatoes right out of the jar, drained, with lemon and salt.

Kangaroo Stew
makes 4 servings

• •
There are no kangaroos in Kangaroo Stew. But as a child, my cousin John liked kangaroos, and when my mom was babysitting him she found that he would happily eat stewed tomatoes with cheese if she presented them to him with a great, kid-friendly name. Don't try this one without home-canned tomatoes.
• •

1 qt. home-canned tomatoes
salt
black pepper
grated cheddar cheese
lemon juice to taste

Heat tomatoes in a heavy, three-quart stainless steel saucepan over low heat. Season to taste with salt and pepper. Stir in grated cheese. It will not melt smoothly. If you would like it to melt smoothly, use American cheese. Season to taste with lemon juice.

My Mom's Slumgullion
makes 4 servings

For years I thought my mom made up this name. Anyone who invents "Kangaroo Stew" should be able to come up with "Slumgullion," right? But it's a real word, probably from Irish Gaelic, and it means a watery meat stew. I don't remember Mom's Slumgullion being particularly watery, but when I consider the other options for this dish, which generally crops up in other cookbooks under ethnically confused names like Goulash or Chop Suey, Slumgullion doesn't sound so bad.

Whatever you call it, it's the most basic meat-tomato-macaroni mixture around. You could add garlic; you could add Worcestershire sauce; but if you keep monkeying with it, at some point, it won't be Slumgullion anymore. My mom said she took a big pot of this up the canyon once for a church function, and everyone gobbled it down.

1 pound ground beef
1 large onion
2 Tbsp. tomato paste
1 qt. home-canned tomatoes
2 cups cooked macaroni
black pepper

grated cheddar cheese

Brown and crumble beef in heavy, three-quart stainless steel saucepan over medium heat. Remove beef and pour off all but 1 tablespoon of grease. Add onion and sauté until clear. Return beef to pan. Mix in tomato paste. Add tomatoes and bring to boil. Add macaroni. Heat through. Season with black pepper and serve with grated cheese. The flavor improves after a few hours in the refrigerator and a quick reheat.

Quick Meals

Sausage, Beans, and Rice
makes 4 servings

• •

Fast and easy, this dish is a great way to stretch a pound of sausage to feed a family. The tomatoes, paprika, and green pepper give a slightly baked-bean taste to the smoky sauce. This is delicious with Classic Cornbread (p. 77).

• •

1 pound smoked sausage, like a Polish kielbasa or a turkey kielbasa, sliced diagonally ¼-inch thick
3 cloves garlic, minced
1 onion, cut into small dice
½ green pepper, cut into small dice
1 tsp. paprika
½ tsp. oregano
¼ tsp. cayenne
1 (8-oz.) can tomato sauce
1 qt. home-canned tomatoes, puréed, or 2 (14.5-oz.) cans commercially canned crushed tomatoes in puree
2 (15-oz.) cans small red beans, drained and rinsed
dash sugar (optional)

hot cooked rice
chopped scallions
sour cream (optional)

In a deep skillet over medium heat, brown sausage on both sides. Remove sausage. Pour off all but 1 tablespoon of fat. Sauté garlic, onion, and green pepper until softened. Add paprika, oregano, and cayenne and sauté until fragrant. Add tomato sauce and puréed tomatoes. Add sausage and beans. Stir well. Simmer, stirring frequently, until desired thickness, 30 to 40 minutes. Add a dash of sugar to taste.

Serve over hot rice, topped with chopped scallions and optional sour cream.

Beef Enchilada Rice

makes 4 servings

This dish has the same flavor profile as Cowboy Casserole (p. 61), but it is much faster to make, thanks to the instant rice. Cowboy Casserole has a richer taste and better-textured rice, but there are times when you have to make compromises. Here is a recipe for those evenings when you need dinner on the table quickly.

½ pound lean ground beef

½ small onion, diced

1 clove garlic, minced

¼ green bell pepper, diced

2 tsp. chili powder

pinch oregano

½ tsp. salt

1 qt. home-canned tomatoes or 2 (14.5-oz.) cans commercially canned
    diced tomatoes

1½ cups instant rice

optional garnishes:

grated cheese

chopped olives

Tabasco sauce

Brown and crumble ground beef in heavy, three-quart stainless steel saucepan. Remove and pour off all but 1 tablespoon of grease. Sauté onion, garlic, and bell pepper until softened. Add chili powder and oregano and sauté until fragrant. Return beef to pan. Mix well. Add salt and tomatoes. Bring to boil. Stir in instant rice. Cover and remove from heat. Let stand 5 minutes. Serve with optional garnishes.

Chili or Navajo Taco Filling

makes 8 servings

● ●
● This is your basic burger and beans chili but with a deeper taste because of the ●
● cocoa and peanut butter. It's good after 30 minutes in the pot, but the flavors ●
● will be smoother and more integrated after a full hour. This is tasty by itself or ●
● you can use it as a good filling for Navajo Fry Bread (p. 76). ●
● ●

2 pounds extra lean ground beef
1 large onion, chopped
4 garlic cloves, minced
2 Tbsp. chili powder
2 tsp. ground cumin
1 tsp. dried oregano
¾ tsp. salt
1 tsp. cocoa powder
1 tsp. Tabasco sauce
1 qt. home-canned tomatoes or 2 (14.5-oz.) cans commercially canned
    diced tomatoes
2 (15-oz.) cans red kidney beans or small red beans, drained and
    rinsed
water
1 Tbsp. creamy peanut butter
2 tsp. cornstarch, mixed with 2 Tbsp. cold water to create a slurry

to adjust seasonings:
Tabasco sauce
sugar

optional garnishes:
corn chips
grated cheddar cheese
sour cream
warm flour tortillas
lime wedges

Brown and crumble beef in heavy, four-quart stainless steel or enameled Dutch oven over medium heat. Remove with slotted spoon and pour off all but 1 tablespoon of grease. Sauté onion and garlic until softened. Add chili powder, cumin, and oregano and sauté until fragrant. Return beef to pan. Add salt, cocoa powder, and Tabasco sauce. Add tomatoes and beans and water to cover. Bring to boil, reduce heat to low, and cover and simmer 30 minutes, stirring occasionally.

Remove lid and simmer uncovered 20 more minutes, stirring occasionally. Stir in peanut butter. Simmer 10 more minutes. Thicken as desired with cornstarch slurry, stirring constantly until mixture boils and thickens.

Serve with optional garnishes.

Meals to Make from Tomato Sauces (pp. 37–44)

Chile Rellenos Crepes
makes 4 servings

My mom's friend Joanne Kjar gave her this recipe, which we have tweaked and retweaked over the years. The genius of the recipe is to combine the flavors of classic chile rellenos—the chile, the cheese filling, and the egg batter—in a way that avoids the step of deep frying, which can be daunting for a home cook. Joanne wraps the chiles and cheese in light crepes, which provide the soft egg flavor as a foil to the tangy sauce and the spicy peppers.

Do not fear the crepes, or as Joanne calls them, "the egg things." They are as easy to make as pancakes, and even if your first few crepes are not an example of Gallic beauty, no one will notice when they are smothered with delicious tomato sauce and bubbling cheese.

This dish is best when made with fresh peppers or peppers you have prepared and frozen for longer storage, but canned peppers will work, too.

1 recipe Mexican Sauce (p. 42)

8 crepes (see recipe on next page)
2 large Anaheim chiles or 1 (4-oz.) can green chiles, rinsed, seeded,
    and cut into eight strips (see appendix)
¼ onion, minced
4 ounces Monterey Jack cheese—2 ounces cut into long, thin rectangles
    and 2 ounces shredded
a little cheddar cheese, shredded (optional but pretty)

optional garnishes:
Sour cream
Cilantro
Chopped green onions
Shredded lettuce

If using Anaheim chiles prepare by broiling until skin is black.
Then place in metal bowl cover with plastic wrap to steam. Peel, rinse,
remove seeds, and then cut each chile into eight strips (add any accumulated chile juice in the metal bowl to the Mexican Sauce).

Make crepes using recipe below. Crepes can be prepared up to two
days ahead and refrigerated, wrapped well in plastic.

Preheat oven to 325 degrees. Spray 6x10-inch Pyrex casserole dish
with cooking spray. Ladle about ⅓ of the Mexican Sauce over the
bottom of the casserole dish.

Place 1 strip of chile, 1 strip of cheese, a sprinkling of minced
onions, and a few spoonfuls of sauce (try to use half the remaining
sauce among the 8 crepes) along the middle of each crepe, roll up and
place seam-side-down in the baking dish. Top with remaining sauce
and shredded cheese, placing in a wide stripe down the middle of the
crepes so the edges will crisp in the oven.

Bake 30 to 40 minutes at 325 degrees, or until cheese is melted and
bubbly and dish is hot through.

Let stand 5 minutes before serving. Serve with any, all, or none of
the optional garnishes.

Crepes
2 eggs
½ cup milk
¼ cup flour
Vegetable oil for greasing skillet

Blend eggs and milk in blender until frothy. Tap in flour and blend until smooth. Pour into wide mixing bowl, cover with plastic wrap, and (if you have time) let rest at room temperature 30 minutes to 1 hour. If you don't have time, don't worry about it. Your crepes will be a little thicker—you may get 7 crepes instead of 8 crepes—and have a few more air bubbles, but they'll still be fine.

Place small Teflon crepe pan or small Teflon skillet over medium heat. When hot, wipe with a crumpled paper towel dipped in vegetable oil, being careful not to burn yourself.

Working over the wide mixing bowl, ladle a few tablespoons of batter onto the hot skillet, swirl pan to coat the bottom, and let excess run back into the bowl. Place back over heat.

When edges look dry, ease the crepe up with a knife at the edge and flip over. When set on the bottom, remove to a plate and cover with plastic wrap. Oil pan with crumpled paper towel between each crepe, and repeat until all batter is used. You should get 8 crepes.

Baked Mexican Puff
makes 4 servings

• •

This is a terrific brunch dish, and wonderful to take to a gathering or to a neighbor because you can put it together ahead of time and refrigerate it up to one day. Bake shortly before you want to serve or to take to your gathering. Baked Mexican Puff has the flavors of Chile Rellenos and the ease of a bread pudding. It's light, browned, and cheesy—like an omelet baked in a casserole dish. A stripe of rich, red Mexican Sauce runs through the middle of the puff with extra sauce served on top to enhance the flavors and colors of the dish.

• •

1 recipe Mexican Sauce, divided (p. 42)
2 large Anaheim chiles or 1 (4-oz.) can green chiles, rinsed, seeded, and cut into eight strips (see appendix)
4 corn tortillas, cut into strips
8 ounces Monterey Jack cheese, grated
¼ cup salsa
4 eggs, beaten
¼ cup milk
¼ tsp. cumin
¼ tsp. garlic salt

¼ tsp. onion powder
paprika

sour cream
tortilla chips
remaining Mexican Sauce

If using Anaheim chiles prepare by broiling until skin is black. Then place in metal bowl cover with plastic wrap to steam. Peel, rinse, remove seeds, and then cut each chile into eight strips (add any accumulated chile juice in the metal bowl to the Mexican Sauce).

Spray 6½ x 8½-inch Pyrex casserole dish with cooking spray. Place half the chiles on the bottom of the dish. Top with half the tortilla strips, half the cheese, ½ cup Mexican Sauce, and all the salsa. Repeat with remaining chiles, tortilla strips, and cheese.

Beat eggs, milk, and seasonings except paprika. Pour over chiles, tortillas, and cheese. Sprinkle with paprika. At this point, you can tightly cover and refrigerate the puff overnight or up to one day before baking.

Preheat oven to 350 degrees. Bake 30 minutes, or until light, puffy, and knife inserted in center comes out clean. While puff is baking, heat remaining Mexican Sauce.

Let puff stand 5 minutes before cutting into squares. Ladle Mexican Sauce on top, then top with sour cream and serve with tortilla chips.

Thin-Crust Pizza
makes 4 servings

The wafer-thin, olive-oil scented crust is crispy at the edges, chewy in the middle, and deeply browned and blistered on the bottom. Make the dough for the crust at least 24 but not more than 72 hours before baking. Even though it makes three 14-inch pizzas, the crust is so light that the entire batch will satisfy only four as a main course. This recipe was adapted from the January–February 2001 issue of *Cook's Illustrated*.

Crust:

½ tsp. sugar

½ tsp. yeast

¾ cup warm water, minus 1 Tbsp., minus 1½ tsp.

2 cups unbleached flour

½ tsp. salt

1/4 cup extra-virgin olive oil

Place sugar and yeast in warm water. Let sit until creamy. Place flour and salt in bowl of food processor fitted with steel blade. Pulse to sift. With motor running, pour warm water through feed tube. Keep motor running and add olive oil. Process until dough forms a ball, about 30 seconds. Remove dough from processor and knead until smooth. If dough seems dry, knead in warm water a teaspoon at a time until smooth.

Lightly oil inside of gallon-sized zipper-lock bag, place dough inside it, and refrigerate at least 24 hours. If you think about it, knead once or twice during that time.

At least three hours before you want to make the pizza, divide dough into three balls and return to refrigerator. One hour before you want to bake, remove the dough from the refrigerator and place baking stone on lowest oven rack. Preheat oven for one hour at 500 degrees. When the stone is ready, place one ball of dough on a large sheet of parchment paper (large enough to accommodate a 14-inch circle of dough). Flatten with hands. Cover dough with plastic wrap (you may need several sheets) and roll to a 14-inch circle. Remove plastic wrap. Trim parchment to one-inch of the circle and slip parchment-backed dough onto baking peel.

Top pizza with ⅓ of the sauce and ⅓ of your desired toppings. Use peel to transfer dough—parchment and all—to the baking stone.

Bake until cheese is bubbling and edges are deeply browned, about 4 minutes in my oven. Remove with peel. Pizza should release easily from the charred parchment.

Discard parchment and place pizza on a wire rack. Allow to cool two minutes. Cut into wedges with scissors.

Repeat with remaining dough balls.

Pizza Toppings:

Sauce (use Pizza Sauce recipe on page 41)

Pepperoni
Mushrooms
Olives
Mozzarella

Because this pizza is so thin, dress it sparingly. Sauce and cheese alone make a nice pizza, but if you like additional toppings, think singles instead of doubles—a few pieces of pepperoni or a few mushrooms or a few olives instead of a loaded pie. Save your extravagant combinations for a deep-dish pie.

optional garnishes:
mesclun green salad lightly dressed with balsamic vinaigrette (particularly good on cheese pizza)
fresh herbs—basil, rosemary, oregano
drizzle of balsamic vinegar

Deep-Dish Pizza
makes 2 large deep-dish pizzas

• •

This is the place for your extravagant combinations of toppings. The crust is rich with olive oil and crunchy with cornmeal. It rises in the oven, so stretch it as thin as possible in the pan. I like pepperoni, mushrooms, red bell pepper, onions, and green olives on my deep dish pizza, but the possibilities are limited only by your imagination.

• •

1 Tbsp. sugar
1 Tbsp. yeast
¼ cup warm water
3 cups flour
1½ tsp. salt
½ cup cornmeal
1¼ cups warm water
¼ cup olive oil

optional toppings:
sliced mozzarella cheese
1 recipe Pizza Sauce, p. 41 (for two pizzas)
pepperoni

mushrooms (slice thinly and cook with a little garlic first)
sliced red bell pepper
sliced onion
sliced green or black olives
grated Parmesan cheese

Proof yeast and sugar in ¼ cup warm water until there is a high, foamy head. Place flour, salt, and cornmeal in the bowl of a food processor fitted with a steel blade. Pulse 10 times to sift. With motor running, add yeast mixture and pour in warm water until dough ball starts to form. Add olive oil and continue to process until dough is smooth and dough ball is cohesive. Let stand in food processor bowl about 10 minutes. Process 10 more seconds.

Oil a metal mixing bowl with olive oil. Scrape dough into oiled bowl and turn to coat top with oil. Cover with plastic wrap and let rise until doubled. Turn dough from bottom to deflate. Cover with plastic wrap and let rise until doubled again.

Preheat oven to 450 degrees. Spray 12-inch round cake pan with cooking spray. Take one-half of the dough and line bottom and sides of cake pan, pushing and dimpling with your fingertips. If the dough will not stretch, let rest 10 minutes to relax the gluten, and try again. Try to make the dough as thin and even as possible.

If making both pizzas at once, repeat with another cake pan. If saving the remaining pizza dough for another day, place the remaining pizza dough in a zippered gallon storage bag that you have sprayed with cooking spray. It will keep refrigerated up to three days and will develop a sourdough flavor.

Line the dough with mozzarella cheese. Top with one-half of the pizza sauce. Add toppings, starting with meat then vegetables and ending with Parmesan cheese.

Bake 30 to 40 minutes, or until the crust is risen and golden brown and the pie is set. Allow to cool 15 minutes before cutting. Cut in wedges and serve.

Bean Enchiladas
makes 4 servings

- Like so many things, homemade refried beans taste so much better than the commercially canned version. I like them with the addition of chopped green chiles. But even plain, the fresh smoothness and savory onion flavor of these beans make a delicious filling for enchiladas. You can use any canned beans, but I like the meatiness of kidney beans here.

bean mixture:
1 Tbsp. shortening
1 Tbsp. chopped onions
1 (15-oz.) can red kidney beans, drained and rinsed
½ cup water
⅛ tsp. cayenne pepper
½ tsp. black pepper
½ tsp. salt

optional additions to bean mixture:
3 Tbsp. chopped roasted peeled green chiles or canned green chiles
1 cup grated cheddar cheese

enchiladas:
1 recipe Chipotle Enchilada Sauce (p. 43)
2 Tbsp. vegetable oil
8 corn tortillas
grated Parmesan cheese
grated Monterey Jack cheese

garnishes:
chopped cilantro
sliced green onions
sour cream (optional)

Preheat oven to 375 degrees. Spray 8x8-inch casserole dish with cooking spray.

Melt shortening in saucepan. Sauté onions. Add beans. Mash thoroughly. Add water. Simmer 5 minutes. Add cayenne pepper, black pepper, and salt and simmer 5 more minutes. Strain through a sieve to remove skins. If desired, mix in 3 tablespoons chopped green chiles and 1 cup grated cheddar cheese.

Put a thin layer of sauce on the bottom of prepared casserole dish. Heat oil in a non-stick skillet over medium heat. Place a few table-spoons of sauce on a plate. Working with one tortilla at a time, dip both sides of tortilla into sauce and fry briefly on both sides in hot oil, turning with tongs. You are just trying to fry the sauce into the tortilla and soften the tortilla. You do not want a crisp tortilla. Remove tortillas to separate plate as they are softened.

Fill the tortillas with the refried beans and a spoonful of sauce. Roll up and place seam-side down in casserole. Top with remaining sauce, grated Parmesan cheese, and grated Monterey Jack cheese.

Bake 20 to 30 minutes, until bubbly and heated through. Let cool 5 minutes before serving. Serve with chopped cilantro, sliced green onions, and optional sour cream.

Goat Cheese Enchiladas
makes 4 servings

Tangy and creamy. Best right out of the oven showered with fresh cilantro and topped with avocado and sliced radishes.

goat cheese mixture:
6 ounces herb and garlic goat cheese, room temperature
2 cloves garlic (There's never enough garlic in herb and garlic goat cheese!)
¼ cup grated Parmesan cheese
2 Tbsp. chopped cilantro
2 tsp. lime juice

enchiladas
1 recipe Chipotle Enchilada Sauce (p. 43)
2 Tbsp. vegetable oil
8 corn tortillas
grated Parmesan cheese
grated Monterey Jack cheese or cheddar cheese

optional garnishes:
chopped cilantro

sliced radishes
sliced avocados

Preheat oven to 375 degrees. Spray 8x8-inch casserole with cooking spray.

Mix goat cheese, garlic, Parmesan cheese, chopped cilantro, and lime juice until soft and creamy.

Put a thin layer of sauce on the bottom of prepared casserole dish. Heat oil in a non-stick skillet over medium heat. Place a few tablespoons of sauce on a plate. Working with one tortilla at a time, dip both sides of tortilla into sauce and fry briefly on both sides in hot oil, turning with tongs. You are just trying to fry the sauce into the tortilla and soften the tortilla. You do not want a crisp tortilla. Remove tortillas to separate plate as they are softened.

Fill the tortillas with the goat cheese. Roll up and place seam-side down in casserole. Top with remaining sauce, grated Parmesan cheese, and grated Monterey Jack or cheddar cheese.

Bake 20 to 30 minutes, until bubbly and heated through. Serve with chopped cilantro, sliced radishes, and sliced avocados.

Eggplant Parmesan
makes 4 servings

• •
• I omit breading and frying the eggplant because it's a lot of trouble and it dis- •
• guises the flavor of the vegetable. This is a nice, autumnal dish to serve with •
• buttered pasta and a crisp green salad. •
• •

1 eggplant, washed well
kosher salt
olive oil
1 recipe Marinara Sauce (p. 37)
4 ounces mozzarella cheese, thinly sliced
¼ cup grated Parmesan cheese

Remove eggplant stem and blossom end and slice eggplant into ¼-inch rounds. Sprinkle on both sides with salt and layer in a colander. Weight with a bowl or zipper bag filled with water. Place colander in sink for an hour.

Preheat oven to 350 degrees. Spray cooking sheet with cooking spray and brush with olive oil. Wipe eggplant with a paper towel. Place eggplant on cooking sheet in a single layer. Spray the eggplant with cooking spray, and turn to coat with olive oil. Bake about 10 to 15 minutes, turn, and bake about 5 to 10 more minutes, or until eggplant is pliable, brownish, and a bit shriveled. You do not want crispy eggplant. You want tender, delicious eggplant. If you have any doubt about whether it's done, try a piece. It should be soft and yielding.

Spray an 8x8-inch pan with cooking spray. Place a single layer of eggplant in the pan, cutting to fit as necessary. Layer with sauce. Layer with mozzarella. Sprinkle with Parmesan. Repeat, ending with Parmesan cheese.

Bake, uncovered, at 350 degrees in the center of the oven for approximately 30 to 40 minutes, or until cheese is bubbling and dish is heated through. Serve with buttered pasta and a green salad.

Chicken Parmesan
makes 4 servings

I love Chicken Parmesan. I even order the fast-food chicken Parmesan sandwiches when it's been too long since the real thing. This is the real thing: crisp chicken, savory sauce, and bubbling cheese. This is even good cold.

4 large boneless, skinless chicken breast halves, pounded to an even
    thickness or butterflied to an even thickness
salt
black pepper
dash cayenne pepper
flour
1 egg, beaten
soda cracker crumbs, mixed with ¼ cup grated Parmesan cheese
1 recipe Marinara Sauce (p. 37)
1 Tbsp. olive oil
1 Tbsp. vegetable oil
4 ounces mozzarella cheese, grated
¼ cup grated Parmesan cheese

Season chicken with salt, black pepper, and cayenne pepper, rubbing well into chicken. Coat lightly with flour, dip into egg, and coat well with cracker-Parmesan mixture. Place on cooling rack to set the coating for 10 to 15 minutes. Preheat oven to 350 degrees.

While chicken is resting, begin heating marinara sauce in a stainless steel saucepan over medium-low heat. Spray shallow oven-proof casserole dish with cooking spray.

Heat oils in large, non-stick skillet over medium heat. Sauté chicken just until coating is crispy and golden, about 3 minutes per side. Transfer to oven-proof casserole dish and bake 10 minutes.

Top each chicken breast with dollop of hot marinara sauce and one fourth of the cheeses. Return to oven and bake until cheese is melted and chicken is cooked through, approximately 8 to 10 more minutes. Serve with additional marinara sauce, buttered pasta, and a green salad.

Casseroles

Cowboy Casserole
makes 6–8 servings

• •

This casserole is also delicious without the meat if you prefer a vegetarian entrée.

• •

1½ pounds lean ground beef
2 ribs celery, diced
½ green pepper, diced
1 small onion, diced
2 tsp. chili powder
½ cup black olives, sliced

3½ cups cooked rice
1 qt. home-canned tomatoes or 2 (14.5-oz.) cans commercially canned
    diced tomatoes
1 tsp. salt
Black pepper
1 tsp. Worcestershire sauce
Tabasco sauce to taste

optional garnishes:
grated cheddar cheese
additional sliced black olives
additional chopped green peppers

Preheat oven to 325 degrees. In a deep skillet over medium-high heat, brown and crumble ground beef. Remove from skillet and pour off all but 1 tablespoon of the grease. Sauté celery, green pepper, and onion until softened. Add chili powder and sauté until fragrant. Stir in beef, olives, rice, tomatoes, salt, pepper, Worcestershire, and Tabasco sauce. Bring to boil.

Spray 13x9-inch casserole dish with cooking spray. Place mixture in dish and bake about 1 hour, or until heated through. Serve with optional garnishes.

My Mom's Meaty Lasagna
makes 4–6 servings

My mom's lasagna is everything you want from beef lasagna; it's rich, sweet, meaty, and full of cheese. If you like sausage in your lasagna, substitute sweet or hot Italian sausage for half or all of the ground beef, and go from there. I like it the way Mom makes it.

sauce:
1 pound ground beef (substitute sausage if desired)
2 Tbsp. olive oil
1 onion, chopped
2 cloves garlic, minced
1 qt. home-canned tomatoes or 2 (14.5-oz.) cans commercially canned
    diced tomatoes

1 (8-oz.) can tomato sauce
1 Tbsp. chopped parsley
1 tsp. sugar
¼ tsp. salt
1 tsp. dried basil

ricotta filling:
15 ounces ricotta cheese
1 egg
2 ounces grated mozzarella cheese
chopped fresh parsley
chopped fresh basil, if available
salt

casserole:
8–10 ounces sliced mozzarella cheese
1 cup grated Parmesan cheese
12 lasagna noodles, cooked, drained, and put in cool water

to adjust seasonings:
salt
additional dried basil
sugar

Brown and crumble beef and optional sausage in heavy, three-quart, stainless steel saucepan over medium heat. Remove heat and pour off fat. Sauté onion and garlic in olive oil until softened and fragrant. Return meat to pan.

Add tomatoes and tomato sauce, 1 tablespoon chopped parsley, sugar, and ¼ teaspoon of salt. Reduce heat to medium-low and cook uncovered until thick, stirring occasionally and mashing from time to time with a potato masher to break down tomatoes, approximately 30 minutes. Add basil. Taste and adjust seasonings.

While sauce is cooking, mix ricotta cheese, egg, 2 ounces grated mozzarella, chopped parsley and basil, if available, and salt to taste. Set aside.

Spray 13x9-inch Pyrex dish with cooking spray. Spread ⅓ of the meat sauce in the bottom of the pan. Layer on three of the noodles and spread ½ the ricotta filling over them. Add ⅓ of the remaining mozzarella on top.

Repeat the process by layering on three more noodles. Spread ⅓ of the meat sauce on top, then sprinkle on ⅓ of the Parmesan.

Layer on three more noodles. Spread on remaining ricotta filling. Then sprinkle on ⅓ of the mozzarella, and ⅓ of the Parmesan.

Layer on remaining three noodles. Spread on remaining meat sauce and top with remaining mozzarella and Parmesan.

Bake 1 hour, or until cheese is browned and bubbly. Allow to stand 15 minutes at room temperature before cutting into squares.

Vegetable Lasagna
makes 6–8 servings

I feel silly giving you a recipe for vegetable lasagna. Doesn't everyone just throw whatever they have in their fridge into the pan? If there are any secrets to vegetable lasagna, I think they are seasoning every ingredient, paying attention to architecture (noodles must be anchored by cheese), and finding a harmonious assortment of veggies. Here I included eggplant, zucchini, and mushrooms, but this lasagna also works well with spinach and roasted red peppers.

I like to use an assortment of cheeses to play up the different flavors of the vegetables, but if all you have is mozzarella and Parmesan, go for it. Veggie lasagna is infinitely flexible. In fact, if you don't like any vegetables in your lasagna, and if, like my mom, you leave them accusingly on your plate, just omit the veggies in the first place and enjoy a cheese-only variation.

Assorted vegetables (I like eggplant, mushrooms, and zucchini)
12 lasagna noodles, cooked to al dente in salted water, drained, and placed in cool water

cheese sauce:
2 Tbsp. butter
1 garlic clove, peeled and minced
2 Tbsp. flour
1 cup milk
1 tiny dash nutmeg (put a dash of nutmeg in your hand; put half of it back in the bottle; use half of what remains in your hand)
¼ cup grated Parmesan cheese

casserole:
1 recipe Marinara Sauce (p. 37)
½ cup grated Parmesan cheese

15 ounces ricotta cheese
2 or 3 garlic cloves, peeled and minced, divided
1 egg
8 ounces mozzarella cheese, grated
finely chopped parsley
finely chopped fresh basil, if available
salt and pepper
3 ounces Swiss cheese, grated

Choose and prepare the veggies that you want to put in your lasagna. If your veggies are firm, roast them first. If they are watery, sauté them first.

To prepare eggplant and zucchini for lasagna, cut them in quarter-inch slices, salt them lightly, layer in a colander, weight with a water-filled bowl, and let stand in the sink for at least an hour. Then wipe off the salty water that will have accumulated on the surface of each slice and place the slices on a baking sheet sprayed with cooking spray and brushed with olive oil. Spray slices with cooking spray and turn to coat with oil. Roast at 350 degrees until tender, turning once, about 20 minutes. Remove from oven and set aside.

To prepare mushrooms for lasagna, I like to trim the stems and peel them. Slice them and sauté them in olive oil with one of the four minced garlic cloves until they are tender and fragrant. Remove from heat and set aside.

Next, make the cheese sauce to top the lasagna. Melt butter in a heavy, two-quart saucepan over medium heat. Add garlic clove and sauté, stirring until garlic is soft and fragrant. Add flour and stir over heat for one minute or until flour smells nutty. Remove from heat and stir in milk and nutmeg until milk is thoroughly incorporated. Return to heat and cook, stirring until sauce boils and thickens. Add ¼ cup grated Parmesan cheese and stir until melted and smooth. Remove from heat and set aside.

Preheat oven to 350 degrees. Spray 13x9-inch baking dish with cooking spray. Spread ⅓ of the marinara sauce on the bottom of the dish and layer on three of the cooked lasagna noodles. Add a layer of cooked eggplant and mushrooms. Sprinkle with ¼ of the grated mozzarella cheese.

Add three more cooked lasagna noodles. Spread on ⅓ of the marinara sauce and the cooked zucchini slices. Sprinkle with ¼ cup of the grated Parmesan cheese. Add three more cooked lasagna noodles.

In a separate bowl mix together the ricotta cheese, two of the garlic cloves, the egg, ½ of the grated mozzarella cheese, and the chopped herbs. Add salt and pepper to taste. Spread over the lasagna noodles.

Layer on the remaining three lasagna noodles. Top with the remaining marinara sauce and the remaining mozzarella.

Spread the cheese sauce over the mozzarella and sprinkle with Swiss and remaining Parmesan.

Bake, uncovered, for approximately 1 hour, or until top is browned and bubbly. Let stand 15 minutes before cutting into squares.

Dinner for a Crowd

Tamale Chicken
makes 10–12 servings

Louise Baughman is my parents' oldest friend—literally: she's 100. Louise served this creamy, mildly spicy dish at a Relief Society luncheon where it was a big hit. The tamales called for are large, fresh or frozen tamales, like Rico's or Lynn Wilson's. If you can't find fresh or frozen tamales, substitute a larger number of canned tamales.

8 chicken breast halves, boneless and skinless
2 tsp. garlic powder
1 tsp. freshly ground black pepper
2 tsp. chili powder
4 Tbsp. butter
1 green pepper, chopped
1 onion, chopped

1 qt. home-canned tomatoes or 2 (14.5-oz.) cans commercially canned
   diced tomatoes
4 large fresh or frozen tamales, cut into ½-inch pieces or 6 to 8 canned
   tamales, cut into ½-inch pieces
1 can cream of chicken soup
8–16 ounces sour cream, or to taste (start with 8 ounces and blend in
   more as desired)
hot white rice

optional garnishes:
sharp Cheddar cheese, very finely shredded
sliced black olives
chopped parsley

Combine spices and rub over chicken. Cut chicken into very small
bite-sized pieces. Melt butter in a deep, non-reactive Dutch oven or
casserole dish. Brown chicken in butter over medium heat in batches.
Remove. Sauté green pepper and onions. Return chicken to dish.
Cover with tomatoes. Simmer uncovered over low heat, stirring frequently, until chicken is cooked through and tomatoes are reduced by
approximately half.

Add tamales to chicken mixture. Warm through.

In a separate bowl combine soup and sour cream. Gradually whisk
into chicken mixture. Warm through over low heat, stirring frequently,
but do not boil (boiling will curdle the sour cream). Ladle over hot
white rice and sprinkle with cheese, olives, and chopped parsley. Serve
immediately.

Company Dishes

Salmon in Sesame Crust
makes 4 servings

• •

I watched a chef prepare this on "Late Night with David Letterman" and decided I had to duplicate it: delicate, sandstone-colored fish crusted with sesame seeds and served in a soup plate with a glistening moat of crystal-clear tomato water. When I researched that crystalline tomato broth, however, I realized that chefs were recommending a tedious approach to its creation: hours of cooking, straining, and skimming.

If you can your own tomatoes, you will have home-canned tomato juice as a fringe benefit. Not only is it delicious as its own beverage, but home-canned tomato juice naturally separates in the bottle, yielding the crystal-clear tomato water necessary to present this showstopper of a dish. There's a way to avoid this phenomenon when you're canning, but I like the clear liquid too much to go to the trouble.

• •

tomato broth:

1 qt. home-canned tomato juice
pinch of salt

optional garnishes:

blanched fresh corn kernels and chopped peppers
halved cherry tomatoes and sprigs of basil

salmon:

1 Tbsp. olive oil
3 Tbsp. sesame seeds (or 1½ Tbsp. white sesame seeds and 1½ Tbsp. black sesame seeds)
4 salmon fillets, trimmed of skin and fat, bones removed with tweezers

Carefully pour the clear liquid from the top of the jar of home-canned tomato juice. Bring clear liquid to a boil and season to taste with salt. You can drink the remaining home-canned tomato juice, or use it in Tomato Juice Whole Wheat Bread (p. 75).

Arrange a confetti of blanched fresh corn kernels and chopped peppers or a few halved cherry tomatoes and sprigs of basil attractively in flat soup plates, leaving room for a piece of fish.

Heat oil in non-stick skillet. Dip one side of each fillet in sesame seeds. If you want a black and white effect, dip half of each fillet in black sesame seeds and half in white sesame seeds.

Place fillet seed-side-down in hot oil. Cook, turning once, until fish is done, approximately 2-minutes per inch of thickness. You can open the non-seeded side of the fish with the point of a sharp knife and peek in to see whether the fish is cooked to your liking.

Put fish seed-side-up in the middle of the prepared soup plates, and ladle around the hot tomato water. Serve immediately.

If you don't have home-canned tomato juice, or want to prepare this with fresh tomatoes, try this method: Start with four large ripe tomatoes and a pinch of salt. Place tomatoes and salt in a food processor fitted with the steel blade. Process for one to two minutes. Strain and discard pulp. Freeze the purée solid. Let thaw overnight at room temperature. Line a fine mesh metal strainer with a wet paper towel. Pour thawed tomato puree through paper-lined strainer. Discard pulp.

Chicken Cacciatore
makes 4 servings

Chicken "hunter-style" has the earthy tastes of mushrooms, peppers, and herbs. I like this over brown rice, but I think it's more traditionally served over pasta. You can make this dish with all chicken breasts or thighs, or you can use a cut-up chicken. If you use a mix of white and dark meat, give the dark meat a 10-minute head start.

Note the trick to firm up the chicken skin without drying out the meat. The quick trip under the broiler won't give you the shatteringly crisp skin of a roasted chicken, but it will help dispel the flabbiness that sometimes affects the skin of a stewed bird.

2–3 Tbsp. olive oil, divided
1 frying chicken, cut into breasts, thighs, and legs (reserve wings and back for stock); divide each breast into two pieces
salt and pepper
1 pound mushrooms, peeled, trimmed, and cut into quarters or eighths (depending on size)

1 onion, halved and sliced
1 sweet red bell pepper, sliced
2 cloves garlic, sliced
¾ tsp. red pepper flakes
2 tsp. chicken bouillon granules
1 cup water
1 qt. home-canned tomatoes or 2 (14.5-oz.) cans commercially canned
     tomatoes
2 sprigs fresh rosemary
2 sprigs fresh thyme
cooked pasta or rice
fresh basil, chopped
grated Parmesan

Heat half of the oil in a deep, stainless steel sauté pan over medium heat. Season chicken with salt and pepper. Place chicken skin-side down in oil and sauté until golden brown, about 4 minutes. Turn with tongs and brown the other side. Remove.

Drain chicken fat from sauté pan. Do not disturb browned bits on bottom of skillet. Heat remaining oil in sauté pan. Sauté mushrooms, onion, bell pepper, and garlic until softened. Add red pepper flakes and sauté until fragrant. Add chicken bouillon granules, water, and tomatoes and bring to boil, scraping the bottom of the pan to deglaze. Return chicken thighs and legs to pan, skin-side up.

Tie a string around the rosemary and thyme to keep them together and make removal easier. Add the herbs and tie the other end of the string around the pan's handle. Remember to trim the end of the string so you don't catch the place on fire.

Reduce heat to medium-low and cover pan. Cook 10 minutes. Add chicken breasts. Cover pan. Cook until chicken is tender, about 20 more minutes.

Adjust oven rack to top of oven and preheat broiler. Place chicken skin-side-up in a shallow, oven-proof pan. Surround but do not cover chicken with cooking juices. Broil to refirm chicken skin, 3–4 minutes. Keep an eye on it. You're just recrisping the skin, not cooking the chicken.

Remove chicken to serving platter. Add juices to tomato-vegetable mixture. While chicken is under the broiler, raise the heat under the tomato-vegetable mixture and reduce to desired sauce consistency, about 8 minutes. If serving over pasta, you can also cook the pasta during this time.

Remove rosemary and thyme. Serve chicken and sauce over pasta or hot rice, garnished with fresh, chopped basil and grated Parmesan.

Breads

Great soup or pasta needs great bread on the side. Only one of these recipes includes tomatoes, but they all pair beautifully with your tomato-based dishes.

Rosie's Quick Baguettes
makes 3 baguettes

The hardest part of making these baguettes is scraping out and washing the food processor. Diastatic malt powder gives the baguettes great taste and texture. You can find it at King Arthur Flour, 1-800-827-6836.

Because these baguettes are designed for those days when you want bread without a lot of planning, they don't call for either a sponge or a starter, both of which enhance the flavor and texture of bread. If you end up making baguettes fairly regularly—say, twice a week—get into the habit of saving a little raw dough (about the size of a walnut) in a plastic bag in the refrigerator and adding it to your next batch. You will be amazed by the boost of flavor.

1 Tbsp. yeast
1 Tbsp. sugar
¼ cup warm water

3½ cups flour
1 Tbsp. diastatic malt powder
1 Tbsp. powdered milk
1½ tsp. salt
1¼ cup lukewarm water

Place yeast and sugar in ¼ cup warm water. Let proof until there is a vigorous head on the water.

Place flour, malt powder, powdered milk, and salt in bowl of a food processor fitted with steel blade. Pulse 10 times to sift.

With motor running, pour in yeast mixture and enough warm water until mixture forms a cohesive ball. It may not completely clean the bowl, but if it is very loose, shake in a little flour and process until a cohesive ball forms. Let stand in food processor bowl about 10 minutes. If very dry, add another tablespoon or so of water. Process about 10 more seconds.

Oil a three-quart metal bowl with vegetable oil. Turn the dough into the bowl and turn again to coat the top with oil. Cover with plastic wrap. Let rise until doubled. Gently deflate. Let rise to double again.

Divide into three pieces. Shape each piece into a rectangle. Working one piece at a time, place rectangle in front of you like a book. Using the side of your hand, form a shallow groove down the middle of the rectangle, like the binding of a book. Fold the short ends of the rectangle into the middle and pinch together. Using the side of your hand, create another groove down the middle, further pinching the short ends of the rectangle together. You should now have a smaller, tighter rectangle. Bring the sides into the middle again, pinch together, and then create another groove with the side of your hand. Repeat one more time, pinching the sides together firmly and tapering the ends to form the classic baguette shape.

Repeat with the other two pieces of dough. This procedure forms the baguettes into tight cylinders, with a "skin" that holds the rise and the shape of the finished bread.

As you shape it, place each baguette onto your baking pan. I use a non-stick, perforated baguette pan from Chicago Metallic. Cover with plastic wrap. Let rise to double.

While bread is rising, preheat oven to 450 degrees. Bake 15 minutes, spritzing with water every 5 minutes. I use a laundry spray bottle filled with clean water. Bake 5 more minutes, then drop heat to 350 degrees for the final 5 to 10 minutes of baking, or until bread sounds hollow when tapped. Cool on racks.

Tomato Juice Whole Wheat Bread
makes 4 loaves

• •
Trust me, the tomato juice in the bread isn't a gimmick; it's actually very good. It gives this dense, chewy bread a slightly sweet and sour taste, which is wonderful with cheese. This makes quite a lot of bread, but the loaves freeze well. To freeze double wrap each loaf in plastic. Let thaw at room temperature before unwrapping.
• •

1 Tbsp. yeast
1 tsp. sugar
⅓ cup warm water, plus 1 cup warm water
1⅓ cup tomato juice
1 Tbsp. plus 1 tsp. salt
⅓ cup honey
2 Tbsp. plus 2 tsp. molasses
2 Tbsp. plus 2 tsp. shortening
6 cups whole wheat flour
1 Tbsp. butter, melted

Dissolve yeast and sugar in ⅓ cup warm water. Add remaining warm water, tomato juice, salt, honey, molasses, and shortening to yeast mixture. Add half of flour and beat until well blended. Add enough remaining flour, cup by cup, until dough is moderately stiff. Knead until smooth and elastic, about ten minutes. Place in oiled bowl, turn to coat. Cover with plastic wrap. Let rise until doubled. Punch down.

Shape into four loaves. Put into well-greased bread pans. Cover with plastic wrap. Let rise until doubled. Preheat oven to 350 degrees. Bake 40 to 45 minutes, or until bottom of bread sounds hollow when tapped. Remove from pans, place on racks, brush tops with butter, and turn on sides to cool.

Navajo Fry Bread for Navajo Tacos
makes 8 servings

Our former LDS bishop Dean Bitter used to invite the teenagers of the ward over to his house for Navajo Tacos. Dean was a friend of my folks and a true Renaissance man. After he retired, he taught high school science and math. He loved Shakespeare. He loved history. He told us the story of Navajo Fry Bread, the base for Navajo Tacos.

Even though it is sometimes thought of as a traditional Native American food, Navajo Fry Bread was created of necessity while the Navajo were imprisoned near Fort Sumner. Cut off from their lands and dependent on unfamiliar and often substandard rations, the Navajo subsisted on bread made from flour, dry milk, and baking powder, cooked in lard.

Navajo Fry Bread is bumpy, crunchy, and chewy, and it makes a nice base for the spicy chili filling and toppings of Navajo Tacos—also not a traditional Native American food. Any leftover bread is good with powdered sugar or cinnamon sugar.

1 recipe Chili (p. 49)

Navajo Fry Bread:
2½ cups flour
½ tsp. salt
1 Tbsp. dry milk
2 tsp. baking powder
1 cup warm water
vegetable oil or shortening, for frying

optional taco toppings:
shredded lettuce
shredded cheese
salsa
olives
sour cream
avocados
radishes

Preheat oven to 200 degrees and line baking sheet with paper towels. Also line a draining plate with paper towels.

Stir together flour, salt, milk, and baking powder. Stir in warm water. If dough is very sticky, add more flour, one tablespoon at a time, until dough is soft but cohesive. Don't knead. Let dough rest 15 to 20 minutes.

Cut dough into 8 pieces. On lightly floured surface, pat first piece of dough into a circle about ¼-inch thick.

Heat 1-inch of oil or melted shortening in heavy skillet over medium heat. Oil should be 350 degrees. Test with a small piece of dough. If it starts to fry immediately, the oil is probably ready.

Pat excess flour off first dough circle and carefully lay into the oil. With tongs, depress the middle so the top is submerged under the oil. Fry 3 minutes, or until the bottom is golden. Turn and fry the other side approximately the same amount of time. You do not need the bread to be uniformly golden. Because the bread is so bumpy and irregular, parts will be darker than others. It's okay to have some of the bread pale and some golden brown.

Drain on paper towels. Transfer to baking sheet and place in oven to keep warm. Pat out and cook remaining dough. When all the bread is cooked, top with chili and serve with shredded cheese, shredded lettuce, and other optional taco toppings if desired.

Classic Cornbread
makes 8 servings

• •

You can dress this cornbread up with chiles and cheese, make it savory by reducing the sugar and adding crumbled bacon, or make it sweet and soft by folding in some chopped fresh or frozen corn kernels. I like the classic version best: crisp-crusted but tender, and lightly sweet, it pairs well with any soup.

• •

1¼ cups white flour
¾ cup cornmeal
¼ cup sugar
2 tsp. baking powder
½ tsp. salt
1 cup milk
¼ cup butter, melted and cooled
1 beaten egg
butter for greasing pan

Preheat oven to 400 degrees. Butter 8x8-inch pan.

Mix dry ingredients. In another large bowl whisk together milk, butter, and egg. Add the dry ingredients and stir just until barely combined. Don't worry about a few lumps.

Spread batter into prepared pan and bake for 20 to 25 minutes, or until toothpick inserted in center comes out clean. Cut into squares and serve.

Crunchy Corn Quesadillas
makes as many servings as you want

• •

Is there anything better with tomato soup than grilled cheese? These quesadillas take the grilled cheese concept to a crunchy new level.

• •

Corn tortillas
Cheddar cheese, sliced

Place non-stick skillet over medium heat. Layer slices of cheddar cheese between two corn tortillas and place in skillet. When cheese begins to melt, turn with spatula. Place slices of cheese on top of the tortilla sandwich. When bottom tortilla is lightly browned and crispy, turn again. Cook until cheese on the outside of the tortilla is crispy. Remove from pan, pat off grease, and cut into quarters with kitchen shears. Repeat as desired.

Pantry Staples

My list of pantry staples won't be the same as your list of pantry staples. We all have our favorite go-to items—things our family eats, things we feel comfortable cooking, things that are fast, things that make us feel better. My go-tos won't be the same as yours. But I know how secure I feel when my pantry is stocked with the building blocks I need to feed my family, and I know how at odds I feel when, instead, I'm facing an ingredient with which I have not yet bonded, like the cans of frenched green beans I keep putting to the back of the shelf.

The idea here is to be able to draw part of your groceries from your own pantry: to regularly use and replenish your food storage instead of hoping against hope that you never have to open the dusty cans of beans in the basement and the 50-pound sack of wheat under somebody's bed. To create food storage that you'll actually use, you need to store what you actually eat—and you need to eat what you actually store.

Try this to get started: For a couple of weeks, save all your food receipts and keep a couple of notes about your meals. That information will give you a good sense of what you actually eat and what would be helpful for you to have on hand. The lists on the following pages are only suggestions.

On the Shelf

* Beef and chicken bouillon granules
* Breakfast cereals
* Canned beans: kidney, black, small red, small white, and so forth
* Canned chipotles in adobo
* Canned coconut milk
* Canned corn and other canned vegetables
* Canned fruit
* Canned green chiles
* Canned or bottled fruit and vegetable juices
* Canned or jarred olives
* Canned soup
* Canned sources of protein—whatever you like: tuna, chicken, and so forth
* Canned tamales in chile gravy
* Canned tomato juice
* Canned tomato sauce
* Canned tomatoes
* Chocolate: baking chocolate, chocolate chips, and good chocolate to eat—which you keep carefully hidden
* Cocoa powder
* Condensed milk
* Condiments
* Corn syrup
* Cornmeal
* Dried beans
* Dried fruit
* Dried herbs: basil, oregano, thyme, rosemary, sage, and so forth
* Dried red chiles
* Dried vegetables (dried corn is particularly tasty)
* Evaporated milk
* Fish sauce
* Flour (White flour has a long shelf life if well sealed; whole wheat flour has more nutritive value but a shorter shelf life—if you don't plan to use it promptly, consider keeping it in the freezer.)
* Honey

* Hot chocolate mix
* Low-sodium beef broth
* Low-sodium chicken broth
* Non-fat dry milk
* Oatmeal
* Olive oil
* Pasta (Whole wheat pasta has more nutritive value but a shorter shelf life. Because heavier sauces go better with chunkier pasta, I try to keep spaghetti, fettuccine, penne, and lasagna noodles on hand.)
* Peanut butter
* Rice (White rice has a long shelf life; brown rice is better kept in the freezer.)
* Salsa
* Shortening
* Spices: cayenne, cumin, garlic powder, black peppercorns, onion powder, cinnamon, cloves, red pepper flakes, red chile paste, and so forth
* Sugar: brown, white, powdered
* Tomato paste
* Vanilla extract and other extracts
* Vegetable oil
* Vinegars: red wine vinegar, white wine vinegar, distilled vinegar, balsamic vinegar, and so forth
* Water: distilled and drinking
* Wheat
* Worcestershire sauce

In the Freezer

* Brown rice or whole wheat flour if you don't use them frequently

* Butter and margarine
* Cheese (Freezing changes the texture of cheese and makes it crumbly, but the difference is not as noticeable if the cheese is going to be melted. It can be a good idea to keep some on hand if you rely on cheese as a protein source, so decide what works best for your family.)
* EggBeaters or other frozen egg product (Fresh eggs are perishable. If you can't get to the store, having EggBeaters on hand can be very helpful.)
* Fruit
* Fruit juice concentrates
* Ginger, lemongrass, lime leaves
* Green chiles
* Ice cream
* Meat and fish (chicken breasts, ground beef—formed into patties and individually wrapped for easy defrosting—sausage, individually quick frozen shrimp, and so forth. Buy on sale, wrap well, label, and use within 3 months.)
* Nuts—nuts go rancid quickly at room temperature but last a long time in the freezer
* Tortillas
* Vegetables
* Yeast—I buy yeast in bulk and keep it in the freezer. Then I can fill a small jar that I keep convenient in the refrigerator.

In the Bins or on the Counter

* Bread
* Garlic
* Onions
* Potatoes and sweet potatoes (Keep these far away from the onions and garlic.)

In the Window

It's lovely to have a few pots of herbs growing year-round. What you want to grow depends on what you use, but basil, parsley, chives, rosemary, sage, and thyme are all easy to grow indoors.

In the Refrigerator

The things you need to buy fresh on a regular basis—milk, eggs, cheese, butter, fresh tortillas, fresh fruit, and fresh vegetables, opened oil, opened condiments. I also keep a small jar of yeast in the refrigerator.

Appendix: Food Storage Notes

Bay Leaves: Fresh bay gives a completely different—and better— flavor than dried bay, and bay trees are easy to grow in temperate climates. In Seattle, Washington, my bay tree grew from a 4-inch seedling to a 5-foot bush in six years. Make sure you are growing culinary bay. Ornamental laurel varieties, also sometimes called bay trees, are not the same thing. You can also often find fresh bay leaves in the fresh herbs section of your supermarket.

Fresh bay leaves freeze very well in a doubled plastic bag.

Beans: I call for canned beans in these recipes to save on time and because tomatoes can interfere with the softening of dried beans. Dried beans are pantry staples, however. To substitute dried beans in any of the recipes in this book, soak them overnight in salted water, drain well, and cook the beans to softness with aromatics and low-sodium broth before adding the tomatoes.

Chile Paste, Red: You can find red, green, and yellow chile paste in Asian markets and a lot of grocery stores. The different colors reflect both different colored chiles and the addition of different spices such as turmeric. They come in small plastic tubs and the paste is sealed inside in a plastic bag. They pack a world of flavor into a very concentrated spoonful. After you have broken the internal seal, place into another sealed plastic bag, put back into the plastic tub, and store in your refrigerator. They last a long time.

Chiles, Dried: Whole dried chiles last a long time and are readily available in most supermarkets. Keep them sealed air- and water-tight in a cool, dark place. To use, reconstitute or toast and grind in a food processor to make immensely fragrant and flavorful chili powder. Good all-purpose chiles to keep on hand are New Mexico and California. I also like Ancho, which tastes something like a spicy raisin.

Chiles, Fresh: Roasted, peeled, and cut into strips, fresh chiles freeze beautifully and are wonderful to have on hand for the winter months. I don't grow my own peppers because they would encroach on valuable tomato space, but I buy Anaheim peppers at the Salt Lake Farmers' Market every summer, roast, peel, seed, and cut them into strips, freeze them on plastic-wrap covered cookie sheets, and then stack them in doubled freezer bags.

I'd like to tell you that I buy a box of peppers and prepare them all at once, but frankly, that would take too much planning, and I'd never get it done. I buy double the peppers I need every week, prepare them all, and put the extras in my freezer, accumulating them throughout the summer in my doubled freezer bags. By the end of a summer full of freshly-prepared Chile Rellenos, Baked Mexican Puffs, Enchiladas, and Tortilla Soups, I have a gallon bag full of roasted, peeled, and sliced green chiles stored for the winter. It is like having Hatch, New Mexico, waiting for me in my freezer.

Garlic: The last garlic I bought in a supermarket came from Argentina, and there's no need for your garlic to be better traveled than you are, especially since garlic is so easy to grow and store.

Plant cloves of garlic point-side-up about four-inches down and six-inches apart in a sunny spot in your garden. Plant in September and mulch the new shoots with straw, leaves, or compost during the winter. In the spring, the garlic will come back. Water regularly, but other than that, don't fuss. One of the endearing things about growing garlic is that it is almost impossible to fail: when the leaves turn yellow and flop over, you have succeeded wildly. Water well the day before you are going to harvest your garlic so the soil will be soft. Loosen gently with a trowel, but be careful not to cut the garlic heads. Pull up your garlic, wash it off with a hose, trim the leaves, and let dry for a few days on paper towels.

Store in a leg of cast-off pantyhose (one with a run), knotting between each head of garlic so you can snip a single head off as you need it. Hang your garlic in a cool, dark, dry place. If growing garlic isn't an option for you, you can also find wonderful, locally grown garlic at farmers' markets and store it as noted above.

Ginger: Ginger freezes very well. You can either place the entire peeled root in your freezer and grate it frozen as needed, or even more convenient, peel the root, cut into chunks, and chop in your food processor. Put in a zip top bag, flatten into a thin sheet, and freeze. Then break off chunks of already chopped ginger whenever you need it.

Herbs: To dry fresh herbs for longer storage, wash them with cool water, pat them dry gently, and place them on cookie sheets on which you have placed cooling racks lined with paper towels. Place the cookie sheets in the refrigerator. Turn the herbs several times over a week or so, until completely dry. Either store in the freezer in doubled plastic bags, or in a dark, dry cupboard in a tightly closed glass jar.

Kaffir Lime Leaves: Many Asian markets sell small packages of fresh Kaffir lime leaves, which add a citrus fragrance and flavor to many dishes. Store Kaffir lime leaves in a sealed plastic bag in the freezer.

Lemongrass: Most Asian markets sell lemongrass in bunches, but it freezes well. Cut the stalks into manageable lengths and seal in plastic bags before placing in your freezer.

Shrimp: Individually quick frozen shrimp last approximately three months in the freezer. Thaw according to package directions before using.

Index

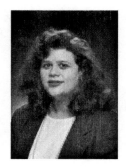

About the Author

Rosemary Reeve is an attorney in Salt Lake City, Utah. She is a graduate of Harvard Law School, a recipient of the Ball Home Canning Award, and a blue-ribbon winner at the Utah State Fair for canned tomatoes. She has been cooking seriously since she was in her teens, when she opened a cookie business to raise money for the building of the LDS Jordan River Temple. She is a frequent speaker on legal topics. This is her first cookbook.